Genuine First Edition Autographed Collectible

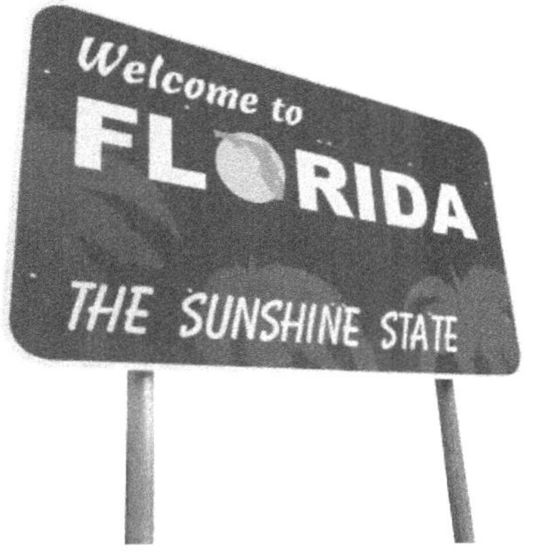

Retirement Planner

It's Never Too Late to Make a **BIG DREAM** Come True!

Date:

To:

From:

Message:

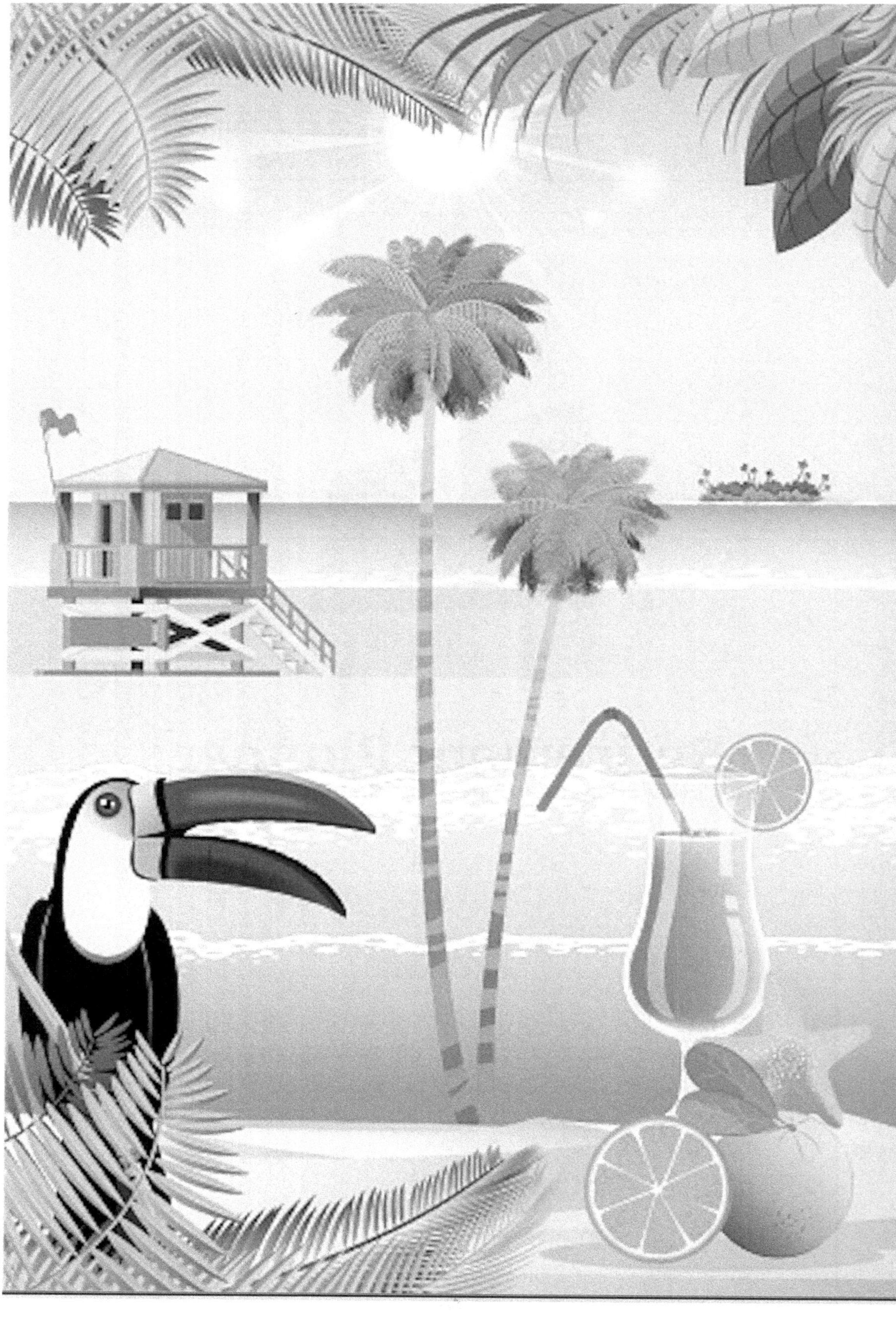

Buried Alive Above Ground in a Florida Condo

How Not to Wake Up, Watch TV, and Wait to Die!

Congratulations!

November 6, 2021
Age 105, Julia "Hurricane" Hawkins, 100-Meter Dash

2021: Age 89, Dr. Manfred Steiner
Earned his Ph.D. in Physics from Brown University.
"Corrections to the Geometrical Interpretation of Bosonization"

Married at Age 95 on May 22, 2021
Joy Morrow-Nulton (age 95) and John Shults Jr. (age 95)
(Both widowed twice after 60-plus years of marriage)

Self-Help, Aging, Health, Gerontology, Retirement Planner, Organizer

Buried Alive Above Ground in a Florida Condo
How Not to Wake Up, Watch TV, and Wait to Die!

Palm Beach Book Publisher books may be purchased for education, business, or sales promotional use.
ISBN Hardcover: 978-1-885872-82-1
ISBN Paperback: 978-1-885872-83-8
Library of Congress Catalog Card Number: 2021902437

Planner Par Excellence — *Created on Jan 26, 2021*
www.PlannerParExcellence.com

Florida Retirement Planner
www.FloridaRetirementPlanner.com

Book Design: Creative Genius Sharon Esther Lampert
Editor: Dave Segal

Publisher: www.PalmBeachBookPublisher.com
Email: Sharon@PalmBeachBookPublisher.com
Phone: 917-767-5843

To Order Book:
Ingram, 1 Ingram Blvd. La Vergne, TN 37086-3629
Phone: 615-793-5000, Fax orders: 615-287-6990

First Edition
Manufactured in the United States of America

Buried Alive Above Ground in a Florida Condo

How Not to Wake Up, Watch TV, and Wait to Die!

Palm Beach Book Publisher
FULL SERVICE: Write, Edit, Publish, Market, Sales

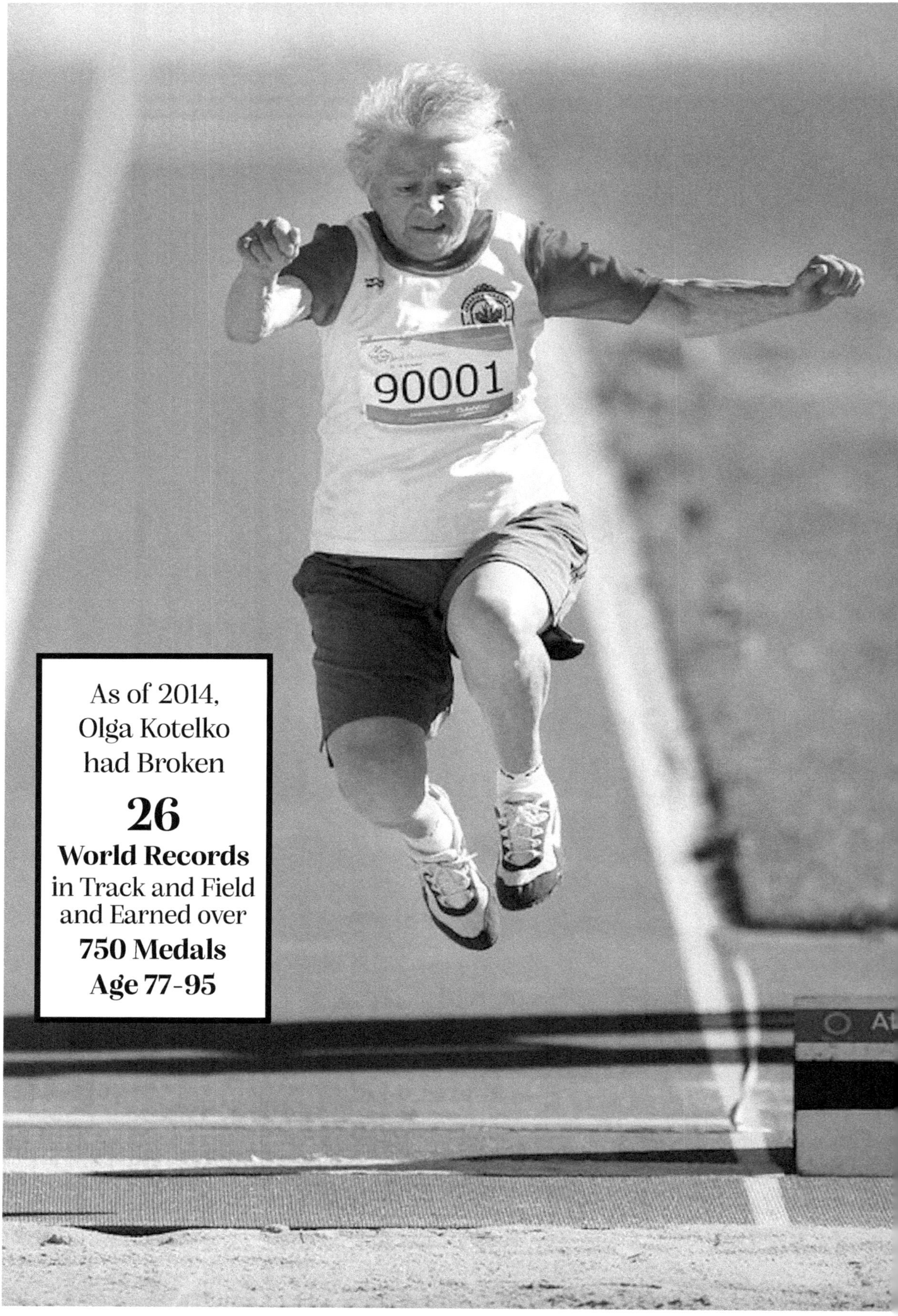

As of 2014,
Olga Kotelko
had Broken

26

World Records
in Track and Field
and Earned over
750 Medals
Age 77-95

Dedication

Olga Marlene Kotelko

750 Gold Medals in Track & Field
Began at Age 77, 80s and 90s
Canadian, 95 Years Old
(Born: March 2, 1919; Died: June 24, 2014)

"I am a warrior, not a worrier and I don't do guilt.

I'm an optimist who moves forward
with focus and determination.

I'm not one of those people who
believes the past is better than the present.

I don't do nostalgia. Everything from our past
eventually fades away after it serves its purpose.

I have discovered that life is meant to be an
adventure, and I haven't come to the end yet!"

For more wisdom from Olga, read her book,

Olga: The O.K. Way to a Healthy, Happy Life

ISBN: 978-1460229446

www.olgakotelko.com

Take Planner Everywhere You Go ...

- Get Organized for a Great Day ✓
- Practice Gratitude and Positive Thinking ✓
- Keep Track of Anything & Everything ✓
- Keep Track of Computer Passwords ✓
- Lose Weight, and Keep the Weight Off ✓
- Never Again Forget the Name of a Book or Movie ✓
- 6 Survival Dating Tips ✓
- 11 Golf Pro Tips ✓
- 8 Tennis Pro Tips ✓
- 28 Games: Card, Board, Groups, and Solo ✓
- Join Digital Revolution on Facebook, Twitter, and ZOOM ✓
- Never Forget a Birthday ✓
- Never Again Forget to Take Your Pills ✓
- Never Again Forget to Apply Sunscreen ✓
- Never Again Forget to Eat Healthy✓
- Never Forget Adorable Things Grandkids Say & Do ✓
- Record Family History Before You Forget! ✓
- Keep Legal Paperwork Up-to-Date ✓
- Travel the Sunshine State ✓
- Make a **BIG DREAM** Come True: Write a Book ✓
- Never Again Forget to Watch a FL Sunrise or Sunset ✓
- Never Again Forget to Look Up for a FL Rainbow ✓

Never Forget Anything Ever Again!

Table of Contents

Introduction p.1

Part 1.
The Planner p.3
DO, DOING, and DONE
7 Shift-Time Management

Facts of Aging Poem by Miriam Gould pp.38-39

Part 2.
The Travel Log, Note Pad, and Journal pp. 41-49

Part 3.
The Organizer p.51

- Retirement: 5-Year Life Transitions p.52
- Mental Health pp.53-55
- Healthy Food Choices p.56
- Lose Weight and Keep the Weight Off p.57
- Computer Passwords pp.58-59
- Doctors & Daily Medications pp.60-61
- Birthday Reminders pp.62-63
- Beloved Grandchildren and the Adorble
- Things Grandkids Say and Do! pp.64-65
- Important Phone Numbers pp.66-67
- Lawyer, Accountant, Financial Advisor, and Banking Information pp.68-69
- 6 Survival Dating Tips p.71
- Favorite Books & Movies pp.72-73
- 11 Golf Pro Tips pp.74-75
- 7 Tennis Pro Tips pp.76-77
- 28 Games: Card, Board, Group, and Solo pp.78-79
- Join Digital Revolution pp.80-81

About the Author pp.82-83
BE BORN poem

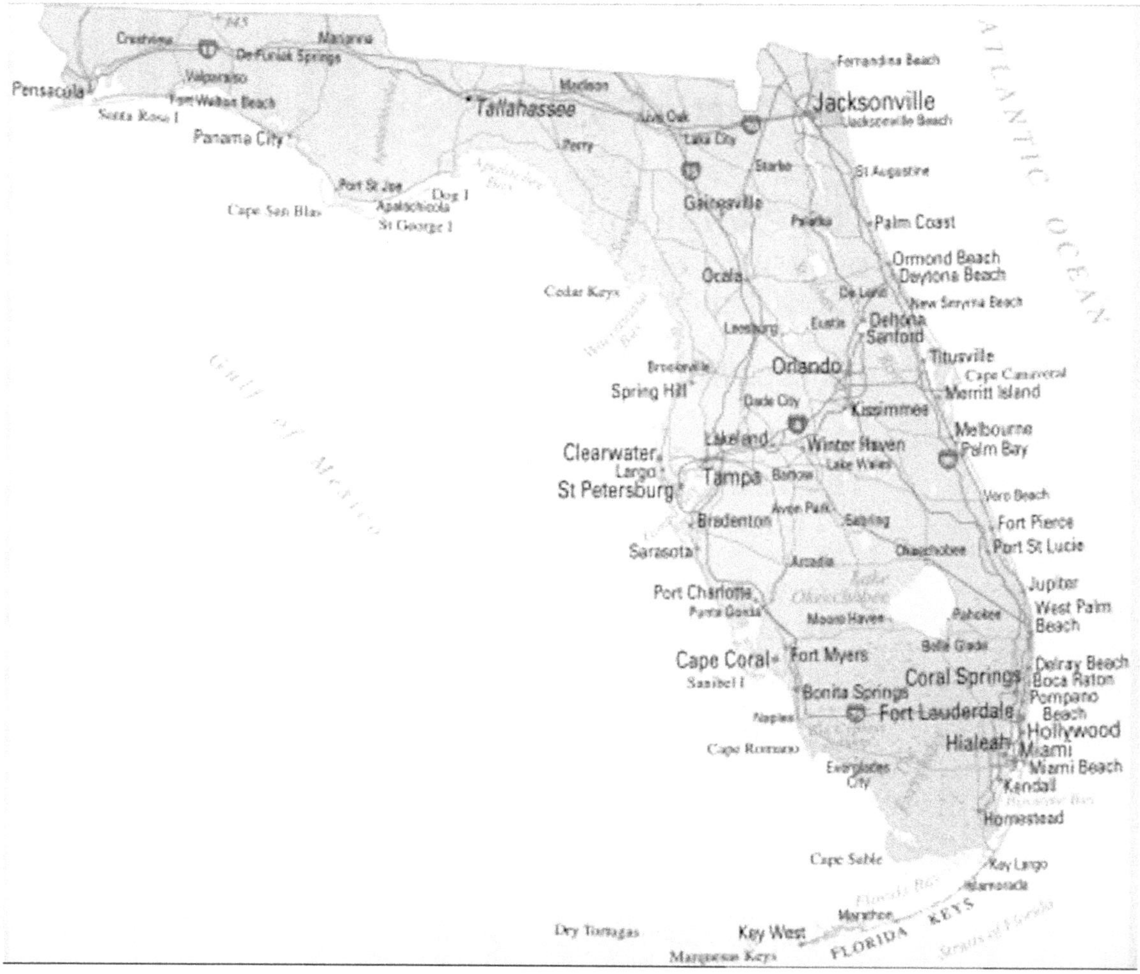

Florida's Most Popular Tourist Attractions:

#1 St. Petersburg: Salvador Dali Museum

#2 Palm Beach: Norton Museum of Art and Sculpture Garden

#3 Orlando: Kennedy Space Center

#4 Florida Keys: Hemingway's House & Dry Tortugas National Pa

#5 Miami: Marlins Baseball Game in an Air-Conditioned Stadium

#6 St. Augustine's Historical District

#7 Boca Raton: Boca Raton Museum of Art

#8 Art Fairs: www.ArtFairCalender.com

Introduction

This Retirement Planner began with a publishing class I taught at a condo clubhouse. My students arrived bearing typewritten manuscripts that were more than 20-years old, and many of them were 85-years of age. Time was not on their side!

At first, I hesitated enforcing a regular writing schedule because retirees no longer want to, or have to, live on a schedule. I was dead wrong!

When I discussed how to divide up the day, and move life's chores to Fridays, or even once a month, and keep the rest of the week open for writing and editing—my students welcomed the structure, discipline, and order.

Soon after, they had transformed from retirees back into college students, and were pulling all-nighters—as they began writing the front and back matter for their manuscripts: dedication, acknowledgements, table of contents, and appendix.

I had completely rearranged their lives, and they were happy to embark on this 6-week publishing journey with me.

The publishing class succeeded beyond anyone's expectations: 5 books were published. The 85+ group were at the front of the lineup!

Esther Tulkoff's memoir, **"I'm Alive Hurray"** was published in less than 6 months, and had become the, "**Miracle Memoir."** At age 86, Esther was able to vividly recall eight decades of her life, and share her joys and sorrows. She wrote her life story on a yellow legal pad, even with her excruciatingly painful arthritis. Esther Tulkoff became a local celebrity with daily book sales of autographed copies: **EstherTulkoff.com.**

—Esther Tulkoff Is an Authoritis!—

I now understand that Retirees want and need a daily structure, so that the day is not wasted by disorganization, chaos, and clutter. This Retirement Planner is the culmination of what Retirees have taught me.

Find a passion, make a plan, and embark on a personal mission. It's never too late to make a **BIG DREAM** come true! Time waits for no one!

Sharon Lampert

Full Service Publisher: Write, Edit, Publish, Market, Sales

Palm Beach Book Publisher: 917-767-5843

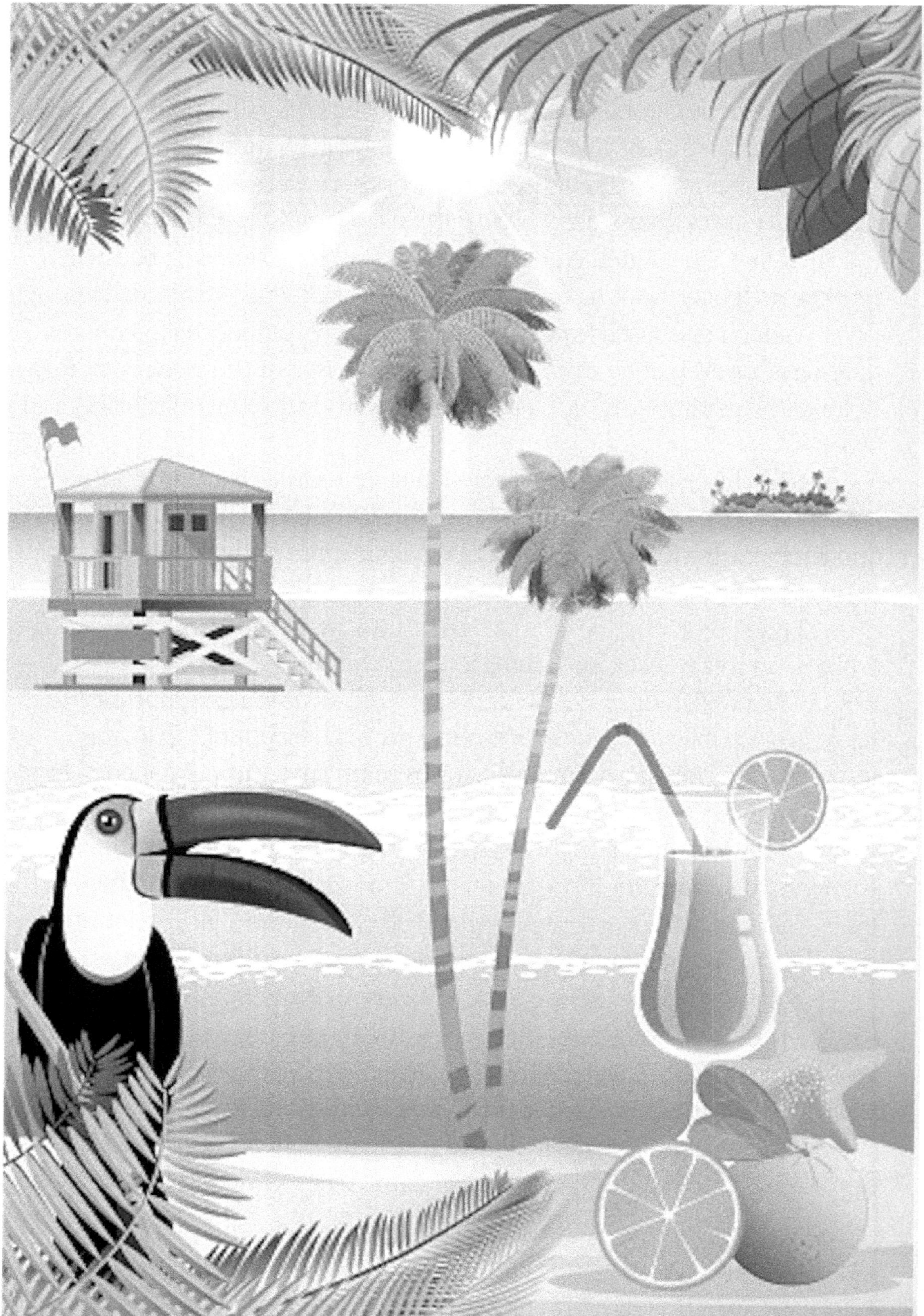

Retirement Planner
It's Never Too Late to Make a BIG DREAM Come True!

Are You an Early Bird or a Night Owl?

The perfect time to start something never arrives

START NOW!

T. Harv Eker

If You Have a PULSE You Have a PURPOSE!

STOP WATCHING THE BAD NEWS!

Bads News Creates Fear, Anxiety, Stress, and Depression, and You Will Be Afraid to Leave the Condo!

The Retirement Planner Helps You Get Started, Stay on Track, and Cross the FINISH LINE!

DO, DOING (DIY or Delegate), and DONE

Practice Daily Gratitude

I am grateful for: ____________________

Practice: "Mindfulness, Meditation, and Mantra Mitigates Madness" S. Lampert
Mantra: ____________________

Healthy Food Choices: Watch Your Weight!

Breakfast: ____________________

Lunch: ____________________

Dinner: ____________________

Snacks: ____________________

Exercise:
Walk, Gym, Tennis, Golf, Swim

____________________ ❑Done

Daily Tasks: DIY or Delegate?

____________________ ❑Done

____________________ ❑Done

____________________ ❑Done

Set Up Restaurant Reservations:

____________________ ❑Done

Phone Calls: Family and Social Life

____________________ ❑Done

____________________ ❑Done

Phone Calls: Business

____________________ ❑Done

____________________ ❑Done

Set Up Doctor Appointments:

____________________ ❑Done

____________________ ❑Done

Free Time—Me Time

Read Book: ____________________

Watch Movie: ____________________

TV Show: ____________________

Travel: ____________________

Night Life: ____________________

Random Acts of Kindness:

____________________ ❑Done

____________________ ❑Done

Household Chores:

____________________ ❑Done

____________________ ❑Done

Run Errands:

____________________ ❑Done

____________________ ❑Done

Buy Stuff or Groceries:

____________________ ❑Done

____________________ ❑Done

____________________ ❑Done

____________________ ❑Done

The perfect time to start something never arrives

START NOW!

7 Shifts: Time Management

Date: ________________

Shift 1. Early Bird: 5-8 A.M.

Shift 2. 9-Noon

Shift 3. Noon-3 P.M.

Shift 4. 3-6 P.M.

My Daily Routine:

- Catch a FL Sunrise ✓
- Check Your POOP! ✓
  Are You Hydrated? ✓
- Bag Pet POOP! ✓
- Appy Sunscreen ✓
  (Behind & Inside Ear!)
- Meditate: Be Here Now! ✓
- Exercise: Walk & Swim ✓
- Eat Whole Foods ✓
- Take Vitamins & Pills ✓
- Call Loved Ones ✓
- Don't Talk About
  Yesterday – Only
  Today and Tomorrow ✓
- Don't Talk About
  Daily Bad News of
  Doom and Gloom ✓
- Open New Chapter
  Pursue a Passion ✓
- Epson Salt Bath ✓
  (Soothes Sore Muscles)
- Catch a FL Sunset ✓
- After Every Rain,
  Catch a FL Rainbow! ✓

Shift 5. 6-9 P.M.

Shift 6. 9-Midnight

Shift 7. Night Owl: 1-3 A.M.

Never regret a day in your life:
Good days give happiness.
Bad days give experience.
Worst days give lessons.
Dr. Sukhraj Dhillon

DO, DOING (DIY or Delegate), and DONE

Practice Daily Gratitude

I am grateful for: ____________________

Practice: "Mindfulness, Meditation, and Mantra Mitigates Madness" S. Lampert

Mantra: ____________________

Healthy Food Choices: Watch Your Weight!

Breakfast: ____________________

Lunch: ____________________

Dinner: ____________________

Snacks: ____________________

Exercise:
Walk, Gym, Tennis, Golf, Swim

____________________ ❑Done

Daily Tasks: DIY or Delegate?

____________________ ❑Done

____________________ ❑Done

____________________ ❑Done

Set Up Restaurant Reservations:

____________________ ❑Done

Phone Calls: Family and Social Life

____________________ ❑Done

____________________ ❑Done

Phone Calls: Business

____________________ ❑Done

____________________ ❑Done

Set Up Doctor Appointments:

____________________ ❑Done

____________________ ❑Done

Free Time—Me Time

Read Book: ____________________

Watch Movie: ____________________

TV Show: ____________________

Travel: ____________________

Night Life: ____________________

Random Acts of Kindness:

____________________ ❑Done

____________________ ❑Done

Household Chores:

____________________ ❑Done

____________________ ❑Done

Run Errands:

____________________ ❑Done

____________________ ❑Done

Buy Stuff or Groceries:

____________________ ❑Done

____________________ ❑Done

____________________ ❑Done

____________________ ❑Done

The perfect time to start something never arrives

START NOW!

7 Shifts: Time Management

Date: _______________

Shift 1. Early Bird: 5-8 A.M.

Shift 2. 9-Noon

Shift 3. Noon-3 P.M.

Shift 4. 3-6 P.M.

My Daily Routine:

- Catch a FL Sunrise ✓
- Check Your POOP! ✓
  Are You Hydrated? ✓
- Bag Pet POOP! ✓
- Appy Sunscreen ✓
  (Behind & Inside Ear!)
- Meditate: Be Here Now! ✓
- Exercise: Walk & Swim ✓
- Eat Whole Foods ✓
- Take Vitamins & Pills ✓
- Call Loved Ones ✓
- Don't Talk About Yesterday – Only Today and Tomorrow ✓
- Don't Talk About Daily Bad News of Doom and Gloom ✓
- Open New Chapter
  Pursue a Passion ✓
- Epson Salt Bath ✓
  (Soothes Sore Muscles)
- Catch a FL Sunset ✓
- After Every Rain, Catch a FL Rainbow! ✓

Shift 5. 6-9 P.M.

Shift 6. 9-Midnight

Shift 7. Night Owl: 1-3 A.M.

Never regret a day in your life:
Good days give happiness.
Bad days give experience.
Worst days give lessons.
Dr. Sukhraj Dhillon

DO, DOING (DIY or Delegate), and DONE

Practice Daily Gratitude

I am grateful for: ____________________

Practice: "Mindfulness, Meditation, and Mantra Mitigates Madness" S. Lampert
Mantra: ____________________

Healthy Food Choices: Watch Your Weight!

Breakfast: ____________________

Lunch: ____________________

Dinner: ____________________

Snacks: ____________________

Exercise:
Walk, Gym, Tennis, Golf, Swim

____________________ ❑Done

Daily Tasks: DIY or Delegate?

____________________ ❑Done

____________________ ❑Done

____________________ ❑Done

Set Up Restaurant Reservations:

____________________ ❑Done

Phone Calls: Family and Social Life

____________________ ❑Done

____________________ ❑Done

Phone Calls: Business

____________________ ❑Done

____________________ ❑Done

Set Up Doctor Appointments:

____________________ ❑Done

____________________ ❑Done

Free Time—Me Time

Read Book: ____________________

Watch Movie: ____________________

TV Show: ____________________

Travel: ____________________

Night Life: ____________________

Random Acts of Kindness:

____________________ ❑Done

____________________ ❑Done

Household Chores:

____________________ ❑Done

____________________ ❑Done

Run Errands:

____________________ ❑Done

____________________ ❑Done

Buy Stuff or Groceries:

____________________ ❑Done

____________________ ❑Done

____________________ ❑Done

____________________ ❑Done

The perfect time to start something never arrives

START NOW!

7 Shifts: Time Management

Date: ________________

My Daily Routine:

- Catch a FL Sunrise ✓
- Check Your POOP! ✓
  Are You Hydrated? ✓
- Bag Pet POOP! ✓
- Appy Sunscreen ✓
  (Behind & Inside Ear!)
- Meditate: Be Here Now! ✓
- Exercise: Walk & Swim ✓
- Eat Whole Foods ✓
- Take Vitamins & Pills ✓
- Call Loved Ones ✓
- Don't Talk About Yesterday – Only Today and Tomorrow ✓
- Don't Talk About Daily Bad News of Doom and Gloom ✓
- Open New Chapter
  Pursue a Passion ✓
- Epson Salt Bath ✓
  (Soothes Sore Muscles)
- Catch a FL Sunset ✓
- After Every Rain,
  Catch a FL Rainbow! ✓

Shift 1. Early Bird: 5-8 A.M.

Shift 2. 9-Noon

Shift 3. Noon-3 P.M.

Shift 4. 3-6 P.M.

Shift 5. 6-9 P.M.

Shift 6. 9-Midnight

Shift 7. Night Owl: 1-3 A.M.

Never regret a day in your life:
Good days give happiness.
Bad days give experience.
Worst days give lessons.

Dr. Sukhraj Dhillon

DO, DOING (DIY or Delegate), and DONE

Practice Daily Gratitude

I am grateful for: ______________________________

Practice: "Mindfulness, Meditation, and Mantra Mitigates Madness" S. Lampert
Mantra: ______________________________

Healthy Food Choices: Watch Your Weight!

Breakfast: ____________________

Lunch: ____________________

Dinner: ____________________

Snacks: ____________________

Exercise:
Walk, Gym, Tennis, Golf, Swim

____________________ ❑Done

Daily Tasks: DIY or Delegate?

____________________ ❑Done

____________________ ❑Done

____________________ ❑Done

Set Up Restaurant Reservations:

____________________ ❑Done

Phone Calls: Family and Social Life

____________________ ❑Done

____________________ ❑Done

Phone Calls: Business

____________________ ❑Done

____________________ ❑Done

Set Up Doctor Appointments:

____________________ ❑Done

____________________ ❑Done

Free Time—Me Time

Read Book: ____________________

Watch Movie: ____________________

TV Show: ____________________

Travel: ____________________

Night Life: ____________________

Random Acts of Kindness:

____________________ ❑Done

____________________ ❑Done

Household Chores:

____________________ ❑Done

____________________ ❑Done

Run Errands:

____________________ ❑Done

____________________ ❑Done

Buy Stuff or Groceries:

____________________ ❑Done

____________________ ❑Done

____________________ ❑Done

____________________ ❑Done

The perfect time to start something never arrives

START NOW!

7 Shifts: Time Management

Date: ________________

Shift 1. Early Bird: 5-8 A.M.

Shift 2. 9-Noon

Shift 3. Noon-3 P.M.

Shift 4. 3-6 P.M.

My Daily Routine:

- Catch a FL Sunrise ✓
- Check Your POOP! ✓
  Are You Hydrated? ✓
- Bag Pet POOP! ✓
- Appy Sunscreen ✓
  (Behind & Inside Ear!)
- Meditate: Be Here Now! ✓
- Exercise: Walk & Swim ✓
- Eat Whole Foods ✓
- Take Vitamins & Pills ✓
- Call Loved Ones ✓
- Don't Talk About
  Yesterday – Only
  Today and Tomorrow ✓
- Don't Talk About
  Daily Bad News of
  Doom and Gloom ✓
- Open New Chapter
  Pursue a Passion ✓
- Epson Salt Bath ✓
  (Soothes Sore Muscles)
- Catch a FL Sunset ✓
- After Every Rain,
  Catch a FL Rainbow! ✓

Shift 5. 6-9 P.M.

Shift 6. 9-Midnight

Shift 7. Night Owl: 1-3 A.M.

Never regret a day in your life:
Good days give happiness.
Bad days give experience.
Worst days give lessons.
Dr. Sukhraj Dhillon

DO, DOING (DIY or Delegate), and DONE

Practice Daily Gratitude

I am grateful for: ______________________________

Practice: "Mindfulness, Meditation, and Mantra Mitigates Madness" S. Lampert
Mantra: ______________________________

Healthy Food Choices: Watch Your Weight!

Breakfast: ____________

Lunch: ____________

Dinner: ____________

Snacks: ____________

Exercise:
Walk, Gym, Tennis, Golf, Swim

____________ ❑Done

Daily Tasks: DIY or Delegate?

____________ ❑Done

____________ ❑Done

____________ ❑Done

Set Up Restaurant Reservations:

____________ ❑Done

Phone Calls: Family and Social Life

____________ ❑Done

____________ ❑Done

Phone Calls: Business

____________ ❑Done

____________ ❑Done

Set Up Doctor Appointments:

____________ ❑Done

____________ ❑Done

Free Time—Me Time

Read Book: ____________

Watch Movie: ____________

TV Show: ____________

Travel: ____________

Night Life: ____________

Random Acts of Kindness:

____________ ❑Done

____________ ❑Done

Household Chores:

____________ ❑Done

____________ ❑Done

Run Errands:

____________ ❑Done

____________ ❑Done

Buy Stuff or Groceries:

____________ ❑Done

____________ ❑Done

____________ ❑Done

____________ ❑Done

The perfect time to start something never arrives

START NOW!

7 Shifts: Time Management

Date: ________________

Shift 1. Early Bird: 5-8 A.M.

Shift 2. 9-Noon

Shift 3. Noon-3 P.M.

Shift 4. 3-6 P.M.

My Daily Routine:

- Catch a FL Sunrise ✓
- Check Your POOP! ✓
  Are You Hydrated? ✓
- Bag Pet POOP! ✓
- Appy Sunscreen ✓
  (Behind & Inside Ear!)
- Meditate: Be Here Now! ✓
- Exercise: Walk & Swim ✓
- Eat Whole Foods ✓
- Take Vitamins & Pills ✓
- Call Loved Ones ✓
- Don't Talk About Yesterday – Only Today and Tomorrow ✓
- Don't Talk About Daily Bad News of Doom and Gloom ✓
- Open New Chapter
  Pursue a Passion ✓
- Epson Salt Bath ✓
  (Soothes Sore Muscles)
- Catch a FL Sunset ✓
- After Every Rain, Catch a FL Rainbow! ✓

Shift 5. 6-9 P.M.

Shift 6. 9-Midnight

Shift 7. Night Owl: 1-3 A.M.

Never regret a day in your life:
Good days give happiness.
Bad days give experience.
Worst days give lessons.
Dr. Sukhraj Dhillon

DO, DOING (DIY or Delegate), and DONE

Practice Daily Gratitude

I am grateful for: ____________________

Practice: "Mindfulness, Meditation, and Mantra Mitigates Madness" S. Lampert
Mantra: ____________________

Healthy Food Choices: Watch Your Weight!

Breakfast: ____________________

Lunch: ____________________

Dinner: ____________________

Snacks: ____________________

Exercise:
Walk, Gym, Tennis, Golf, Swim

____________________ ❑Done

Daily Tasks: DIY or Delegate?

____________________ ❑Done

____________________ ❑Done

____________________ ❑Done

Set Up Restaurant Reservations:

____________________ ❑Done

Phone Calls: Family and Social Life

____________________ ❑Done

____________________ ❑Done

Phone Calls: Business

____________________ ❑Done

____________________ ❑Done

Set Up Doctor Appointments:

____________________ ❑Done

____________________ ❑Done

Free Time—Me Time

Read Book: ____________________

Watch Movie: ____________________

TV Show: ____________________

Travel: ____________________

Night Life: ____________________

Random Acts of Kindness:

____________________ ❑Done

____________________ ❑Done

Household Chores:

____________________ ❑Done

____________________ ❑Done

Run Errands:

____________________ ❑Done

____________________ ❑Done

Buy Stuff or Groceries:

____________________ ❑Done

____________________ ❑Done

____________________ ❑Done

____________________ ❑Done

The perfect time to start something never arrives

START NOW!

7 Shifts: Time Management

Date: ________________

Shift 1. Early Bird: 5-8 A.M.

Shift 2. 9-Noon

Shift 3. Noon-3 P.M.

Shift 4. 3-6 P.M.

My Daily Routine:

- Catch a FL Sunrise ✓
- Check Your POOP! ✓
  Are You Hydrated? ✓
- Bag Pet POOP! ✓
- Appy Sunscreen ✓
  (Behind & Inside Ear!)
- Meditate: Be Here Now! ✓
- Exercise: Walk & Swim ✓
- Eat Whole Foods ✓
- Take Vitamins & Pills ✓
- Call Loved Ones ✓
- Don't Talk About Yesterday – Only Today and Tomorrow ✓
- Don't Talk About Daily Bad News of Doom and Gloom ✓
- Open New Chapter
  Pursue a Passion ✓
- Epson Salt Bath ✓
  (Soothes Sore Muscles)
- Catch a FL Sunset ✓
- After Every Rain, Catch a FL Rainbow! ✓

Shift 5. 6-9 P.M.

Shift 6. 9-Midnight

Shift 7. Night Owl: 1-3 A.M.

Never regret a day in your life:
Good days give happiness.
Bad days give experience.
Worst days give lessons.
Dr. Sukhraj Dhillon

DO, DOING (DIY or Delegate), and DONE

Practice Daily Gratitude

I am grateful for: ______________________________

Practice: "Mindfulness, Meditation, and Mantra Mitigates Madness" S. Lampert
Mantra: ______________________________

Healthy Food Choices: Watch Your Weight!

Breakfast: ____________________

Lunch: ____________________

Dinner: ____________________

Snacks: ____________________

Exercise:
Walk, Gym, Tennis, Golf, Swim

____________________ ❑Done

Daily Tasks: DIY or Delegate?

____________________ ❑Done

____________________ ❑Done

____________________ ❑Done

Set Up Restaurant Reservations:

____________________ ❑Done

Phone Calls: Family and Social Life

____________________ ❑Done

____________________ ❑Done

Phone Calls: Business

____________________ ❑Done

____________________ ❑Done

Set Up Doctor Appointments:

____________________ ❑Done

____________________ ❑Done

Free Time—Me Time

Read Book: ____________________

Watch Movie: ____________________

TV Show: ____________________

Travel: ____________________

Night Life: ____________________

Random Acts of Kindness:

____________________ ❑Done

____________________ ❑Done

Household Chores:

____________________ ❑Done

____________________ ❑Done

Run Errands:

____________________ ❑Done

____________________ ❑Done

Buy Stuff or Groceries:

____________________ ❑Done

____________________ ❑Done

____________________ ❑Done

____________________ ❑Done

The perfect time to start something never arrives

START NOW!

7 Shifts: Time Management

Date: ________________

Shift 1. Early Bird: 5-8 A.M.

Shift 2. 9-Noon

Shift 3. Noon-3 P.M.

Shift 4. 3-6 P.M.

My Daily Routine:

- Catch a FL Sunrise ✓
- Check Your POOP! ✓
  Are You Hydrated? ✓
- Bag Pet POOP! ✓
- Appy Sunscreen ✓
  (Behind & Inside Ear!)
- Meditate: Be Here Now! ✓
- Exercise: Walk & Swim ✓
- Eat Whole Foods ✓
- Take Vitamins & Pills ✓
- Call Loved Ones ✓
- Don't Talk About Yesterday – Only Today and Tomorrow ✓
- Don't Talk About Daily Bad News of Doom and Gloom ✓
- Open New Chapter
  Pursue a Passion ✓
- Epson Salt Bath ✓
  (Soothes Sore Muscles)
- Catch a FL Sunset ✓
- After Every Rain, Catch a FL Rainbow! ✓

Shift 5. 6-9 P.M.

Shift 6. 9-Midnight

Shift 7. Night Owl: 1-3 A.M.

Never regret a day in your life:
Good days give happiness.
Bad days give experience.
Worst days give lessons.
Dr. Sukhraj Dhillon

DO, DOING (DIY or Delegate), and DONE

Practice Daily Gratitude

I am grateful for: ____________________

Practice: "Mindfulness, Meditation, and Mantra Mitigates Madness" S. Lampert
Mantra: ____________________

Healthy Food Choices: Watch Your Weight!

Breakfast: ____________________

Lunch: ____________________

Dinner: ____________________

Snacks: ____________________

Exercise:
Walk, Gym, Tennis, Golf, Swim

____________________ ❑Done

Daily Tasks: DIY or Delegate?

____________________ ❑Done

____________________ ❑Done

____________________ ❑Done

Set Up Restaurant Reservations:

____________________ ❑Done

Phone Calls: Family and Social Life

____________________ ❑Done

____________________ ❑Done

Phone Calls: Business

____________________ ❑Done

____________________ ❑Done

Set Up Doctor Appointments:

____________________ ❑Done

____________________ ❑Done

Free Time—Me Time

Read Book: ____________________

Watch Movie: ____________________

TV Show: ____________________

Travel: ____________________

Night Life: ____________________

Random Acts of Kindness:

____________________ ❑Done

____________________ ❑Done

Household Chores:

____________________ ❑Done

____________________ ❑Done

Run Errands:

____________________ ❑Done

____________________ ❑Done

Buy Stuff or Groceries:

____________________ ❑Done

____________________ ❑Done

____________________ ❑Done

____________________ ❑Done

The perfect time to start something never arrives

START NOW!

7 Shifts: Time Management

Date: ________________

Shift 1. Early Bird: 5-8 A.M.

Shift 2. 9-Noon

Shift 3. Noon-3 P.M.

Shift 4. 3-6 P.M.

My Daily Routine:

- Catch a FL Sunrise ✓
- Check Your POOP! ✓
  Are You Hydrated? ✓
- Bag Pet POOP! ✓
- Appy Sunscreen ✓
  (Behind & Inside Ear!)
- Meditate: Be Here Now! ✓
- Exercise: Walk & Swim ✓
- Eat Whole Foods ✓
- Take Vitamins & Pills ✓
- Call Loved Ones ✓
- Don't Talk About Yesterday – Only Today and Tomorrow ✓
- Don't Talk About Daily Bad News of Doom and Gloom ✓
- Open New Chapter
  Pursue a Passion ✓
- Epson Salt Bath ✓
  (Soothes Sore Muscles)
- Catch a FL Sunset ✓
- After Every Rain, Catch a FL Rainbow! ✓

Shift 5. 6-9 P.M.

Shift 6. 9-Midnight

Shift 7. Night Owl: 1-3 A.M.

Never regret a day in your life:
Good days give happiness.
Bad days give experience.
Worst days give lessons.
Dr. Sukhraj Dhillon

DO, DOING (DIY or Delegate), and DONE

Practice Daily Gratitude

I am grateful for: ____________________

Practice: "Mindfulness, Meditation, and Mantra Mitigates Madness" S. Lampert
Mantra: ____________________

Healthy Food Choices: Watch Your Weight!

Breakfast: ____________________

Lunch: ____________________

Dinner: ____________________

Snacks: ____________________

Exercise:
Walk, Gym, Tennis, Golf, Swim

____________________ ❑Done

Daily Tasks: DIY or Delegate?

____________________ ❑Done

____________________ ❑Done

____________________ ❑Done

Set Up Restaurant Reservations:

____________________ ❑Done

Phone Calls: Family and Social Life

____________________ ❑Done

____________________ ❑Done

Phone Calls: Business

____________________ ❑Done

____________________ ❑Done

Set Up Doctor Appointments:

____________________ ❑Done

____________________ ❑Done

Free Time—Me Time

Read Book: ____________________

Watch Movie: ____________________

TV Show: ____________________

Travel: ____________________

Night Life: ____________________

Random Acts of Kindness:

____________________ ❑Done

____________________ ❑Done

Household Chores:

____________________ ❑Done

____________________ ❑Done

Run Errands:

____________________ ❑Done

____________________ ❑Done

Buy Stuff or Groceries:

____________________ ❑Done

____________________ ❑Done

____________________ ❑Done

____________________ ❑Done

The perfect time to start something never arrives

START NOW!

7 Shifts: Time Management

Date: ________________

Shift 1. Early Bird: 5-8 A.M.

Shift 2. 9-Noon

Shift 3. Noon-3 P.M.

Shift 4. 3-6 P.M.

My Daily Routine:

- Catch a FL Sunrise ✓
- Check Your POOP! ✓
  Are You Hydrated? ✓
- Bag Pet POOP! ✓
- Appy Sunscreen ✓
  (Behind & Inside Ear!)
- Meditate: Be Here Now! ✓
- Exercise: Walk & Swim ✓
- Eat Whole Foods ✓
- Take Vitamins & Pills ✓
- Call Loved Ones ✓
- Don't Talk About Yesterday – Only Today and Tomorrow ✓
- Don't Talk About Daily Bad News of Doom and Gloom ✓
- Open New Chapter
  Pursue a Passion ✓
- Epson Salt Bath ✓
  (Soothes Sore Muscles)
- Catch a FL Sunset ✓
- After Every Rain, Catch a FL Rainbow! ✓

Shift 5. 6-9 P.M.

Shift 6. 9-Midnight

Shift 7. Night Owl: 1-3 A.M.

Never regret a day in your life:
Good days give happiness.
Bad days give experience.
Worst days give lessons.
Dr. Sukhraj Dhillon

DO, DOING (DIY or Delegate), and DONE

Practice Daily Gratitude

I am grateful for: ____________________________

Practice: "Mindfulness, Meditation, and Mantra Mitigates Madness" S. Lampert
Mantra: ____________________________

Healthy Food Choices: Watch Your Weight!

Breakfast: ____________________

Lunch: ____________________

Dinner: ____________________

Snacks: ____________________

Exercise:
Walk, Gym, Tennis, Golf, Swim

____________________ ❑Done

Daily Tasks: DIY or Delegate?

____________________ ❑Done

____________________ ❑Done

____________________ ❑Done

Set Up Restaurant Reservations:

____________________ ❑Done

Phone Calls: Family and Social Life

____________________ ❑Done

____________________ ❑Done

Phone Calls: Business

____________________ ❑Done

____________________ ❑Done

Set Up Doctor Appointments:

____________________ ❑Done

____________________ ❑Done

Free Time—Me Time

Read Book: ____________________

Watch Movie: ____________________

TV Show: ____________________

Travel: ____________________

Night Life: ____________________

Random Acts of Kindness:

____________________ ❑Done

____________________ ❑Done

Household Chores:

____________________ ❑Done

____________________ ❑Done

Run Errands:

____________________ ❑Done

____________________ ❑Done

Buy Stuff or Groceries:

____________________ ❑Done

____________________ ❑Done

____________________ ❑Done

____________________ ❑Done

The perfect time to start something never arrives

START NOW!

7 Shifts: Time Management

Date: ________________

Shift 1. Early Bird: 5-8 A.M.

Shift 2. 9-Noon

Shift 3. Noon-3 P.M.

Shift 4. 3-6 P.M.

My Daily Routine:

- Catch a FL Sunrise ✓
- Check Your POOP! ✓
  Are You Hydrated? ✓
- Bag Pet POOP! ✓
- Appy Sunscreen ✓
  (Behind & Inside Ear!)
- Meditate: Be Here Now! ✓
- Exercise: Walk & Swim ✓
- Eat Whole Foods ✓
- Take Vitamins & Pills ✓
- Call Loved Ones ✓
- Don't Talk About
  Yesterday – Only
  Today and Tomorrow ✓
- Don't Talk About
  Daily Bad News of
  Doom and Gloom ✓
- Open New Chapter
  Pursue a Passion ✓
- Epson Salt Bath ✓
  (Soothes Sore Muscles)
- Catch a FL Sunset ✓
- After Every Rain,
  Catch a FL Rainbow! ✓

Shift 5. 6-9 P.M.

Shift 6. 9-Midnight

Shift 7. Night Owl: 1-3 A.M.

Never regret a day in your life:
Good days give happiness.
Bad days give experience.
Worst days give lessons.
Dr. Sukhraj Dhillon

DO, DOING (DIY or Delegate), and DONE

Practice Daily Gratitude

I am grateful for: ______________________________

Practice: "Mindfulness, Meditation, and Mantra Mitigates Madness" S. Lampert
Mantra: ______________________________

Healthy Food Choices: Watch Your Weight!

Breakfast: ______________

Lunch: ______________

Dinner: ______________

Snacks: ______________

Exercise:
Walk, Gym, Tennis, Golf, Swim

______________ ❑Done

Daily Tasks: DIY or Delegate?

______________ ❑Done

______________ ❑Done

______________ ❑Done

Set Up Restaurant Reservations:

______________ ❑Done

Phone Calls: Family and Social Life

______________ ❑Done

______________ ❑Done

Phone Calls: Business

______________ ❑Done

______________ ❑Done

Set Up Doctor Appointments:

______________ ❑Done

______________ ❑Done

Free Time—Me Time

Read Book: ______________

Watch Movie: ______________

TV Show: ______________

Travel: ______________

Night Life: ______________

Random Acts of Kindness:

______________ ❑Done

______________ ❑Done

Household Chores:

______________ ❑Done

______________ ❑Done

Run Errands:

______________ ❑Done

______________ ❑Done

Buy Stuff or Groceries:

______________ ❑Done

______________ ❑Done

______________ ❑Done

______________ ❑Done

The perfect time to start something never arrives

START NOW!

7 Shifts: Time Management

Date: _______________

Shift 1. Early Bird: 5-8 A.M.

Shift 2. 9-Noon

Shift 3. Noon-3 P.M.

Shift 4. 3-6 P.M.

My Daily Routine:

- Catch a FL Sunrise ✓
- Check Your POOP! ✓
  Are You Hydrated? ✓
- Bag Pet POOP! ✓
- Appy Sunscreen ✓
  (Behind & Inside Ear!)
- Meditate: Be Here Now! ✓
- Exercise: Walk & Swim ✓
- Eat Whole Foods ✓
- Take Vitamins & Pills ✓
- Call Loved Ones ✓
- Don't Talk About Yesterday – Only Today and Tomorrow ✓
- Don't Talk About Daily Bad News of Doom and Gloom ✓
- Open New Chapter
  Pursue a Passion ✓
- Epson Salt Bath ✓
  (Soothes Sore Muscles)
- Catch a FL Sunset ✓
- After Every Rain,
  Catch a FL Rainbow! ✓

Shift 5. 6-9 P.M.

Shift 6. 9-Midnight

Shift 7. Night Owl: 1-3 A.M.

Never regret a day in your life:
Good days give happiness.
Bad days give experience.
Worst days give lessons.
Dr. Sukhraj Dhillon

DO, DOING (DIY or Delegate), and DONE

Practice Daily Gratitude

I am grateful for: ______________________________

Practice: "Mindfulness, Meditation, and Mantra Mitigates Madness" S. Lampert
Mantra: ______________________________

Healthy Food Choices: Watch Your Weight!

Breakfast: ____________________

Lunch: ____________________

Dinner: ____________________

Snacks: ____________________

Exercise:
Walk, Gym, Tennis, Golf, Swim

____________________ ❑Done

Daily Tasks: DIY or Delegate?

____________________ ❑Done

____________________ ❑Done

____________________ ❑Done

Set Up Restaurant Reservations:

____________________ ❑Done

Phone Calls: Family and Social Life

____________________ ❑Done

____________________ ❑Done

Phone Calls: Business

____________________ ❑Done

____________________ ❑Done

Set Up Doctor Appointments:

____________________ ❑Done

____________________ ❑Done

Free Time—Me Time

Read Book: ____________________

Watch Movie: ____________________

TV Show: ____________________

Travel: ____________________

Night Life: ____________________

Random Acts of Kindness:

____________________ ❑Done

____________________ ❑Done

Household Chores:

____________________ ❑Done

____________________ ❑Done

Run Errands:

____________________ ❑Done

____________________ ❑Done

Buy Stuff or Groceries:

____________________ ❑Done

____________________ ❑Done

____________________ ❑Done

____________________ ❑Done

The perfect time to start something never arrives

START NOW!

7 Shifts: Time Management

Date: ________________

Shift 1. Early Bird: 5-8 A.M.

Shift 2. 9-Noon

Shift 3. Noon-3 P.M.

Shift 4. 3-6 P.M.

My Daily Routine:

- Catch a FL Sunrise ✓
- Check Your POOP! ✓
  Are You Hydrated? ✓
- Bag Pet POOP! ✓
- Appy Sunscreen ✓
  (Behind & Inside Ear!)
- Meditate: Be Here Now! ✓
- Exercise: Walk & Swim ✓
- Eat Whole Foods ✓
- Take Vitamins & Pills ✓
- Call Loved Ones ✓
- Don't Talk About Yesterday – Only Today and Tomorrow ✓
- Don't Talk About Daily Bad News of Doom and Gloom ✓
- Open New Chapter
  Pursue a Passion ✓
- Epson Salt Bath ✓
  (Soothes Sore Muscles)
- Catch a FL Sunset ✓
- After Every Rain, Catch a FL Rainbow! ✓

Shift 5. 6-9 P.M.

Shift 6. 9-Midnight

Shift 7. Night Owl: 1-3 A.M.

Never regret a day in your life:
Good days give happiness.
Bad days give experience.
Worst days give lessons.
Dr. Sukhraj Dhillon

DO, DOING (DIY or Delegate), and DONE

Practice Daily Gratitude

I am grateful for: ____________________

Practice: "Mindfulness, Meditation, and Mantra Mitigates Madness" S. Lampert
Mantra: ____________________

Healthy Food Choices: Watch Your Weight!

Breakfast: ____________________

Lunch: ____________________

Dinner: ____________________

Snacks: ____________________

Exercise:
Walk, Gym, Tennis, Golf, Swim

____________________ ❑Done

Daily Tasks: DIY or Delegate?

____________________ ❑Done

____________________ ❑Done

____________________ ❑Done

Set Up Restaurant Reservations:

____________________ ❑Done

Phone Calls: Family and Social Life

____________________ ❑Done

____________________ ❑Done

Phone Calls: Business

____________________ ❑Done

____________________ ❑Done

Set Up Doctor Appointments:

____________________ ❑Done

____________________ ❑Done

Free Time—Me Time

Read Book: ____________________

Watch Movie: ____________________

TV Show: ____________________

Travel: ____________________

Night Life: ____________________

Random Acts of Kindness:

____________________ ❑Done

____________________ ❑Done

Household Chores:

____________________ ❑Done

____________________ ❑Done

Run Errands:

____________________ ❑Done

____________________ ❑Done

Buy Stuff or Groceries:

____________________ ❑Done

____________________ ❑Done

____________________ ❑Done

____________________ ❑Done

The perfect time to start something never arrives

START NOW!

7 Shifts: Time Management

Date: ________________

Shift 1. Early Bird: 5-8 A.M.

Shift 2. 9-Noon

Shift 3. Noon-3 P.M.

Shift 4. 3-6 P.M.

My Daily Routine:

- Catch a FL Sunrise ✓
- Check Your POOP! ✓
  Are You Hydrated? ✓
- Bag Pet POOP! ✓
- Appy Sunscreen ✓
  (Behind & Inside Ear!)
- Meditate: Be Here Now! ✓
- Exercise: Walk & Swim ✓
- Eat Whole Foods ✓
- Take Vitamins & Pills ✓
- Call Loved Ones ✓
- Don't Talk About Yesterday – Only Today and Tomorrow ✓
- Don't Talk About Daily Bad News of Doom and Gloom ✓
- Open New Chapter
  Pursue a Passion ✓
- Epson Salt Bath ✓
  (Soothes Sore Muscles)
- Catch a FL Sunset ✓
- After Every Rain, Catch a FL Rainbow! ✓

Shift 5. 6-9 P.M.

Shift 6. 9-Midnight

Shift 7. Night Owl: 1-3 A.M.

Never regret a day in your life:
Good days give happiness.
Bad days give experience.
Worst days give lessons.

Dr. Sukhraj Dhillon

DO, DOING (DIY or Delegate), and DONE

Practice Daily Gratitude

I am grateful for: ____________________

Practice: "Mindfulness, Meditation, and Mantra Mitigates Madness" S. Lampert
Mantra: ____________________

Healthy Food Choices: Watch Your Weight!

Breakfast: ____________

Lunch: ____________

Dinner: ____________

Snacks: ____________

Exercise:
Walk, Gym, Tennis, Golf, Swim

____________ ❑Done

Daily Tasks: DIY or Delegate?

____________ ❑Done

____________ ❑Done

____________ ❑Done

Set Up Restaurant Reservations:

____________ ❑Done

Phone Calls: Family and Social Life

____________ ❑Done

____________ ❑Done

Phone Calls: Business

____________ ❑Done

____________ ❑Done

Set Up Doctor Appointments:

____________ ❑Done

____________ ❑Done

Free Time—Me Time

Read Book: ____________

Watch Movie: ____________

TV Show: ____________

Travel: ____________

Night Life: ____________

Random Acts of Kindness:

____________ ❑Done

____________ ❑Done

Household Chores:

____________ ❑Done

____________ ❑Done

Run Errands:

____________ ❑Done

____________ ❑Done

Buy Stuff or Groceries:

____________ ❑Done

____________ ❑Done

____________ ❑Done

____________ ❑Done

The perfect time to start something never arrives

START NOW!

7 Shifts: Time Management

Date: ________________

Shift 1. Early Bird: 5-8 A.M.

Shift 2. 9-Noon

Shift 3. Noon-3 P.M.

Shift 4. 3-6 P.M.

My Daily Routine:

- Catch a FL Sunrise ✓
- Check Your POOP! ✓
  Are You Hydrated? ✓
- Bag Pet POOP! ✓
- Appy Sunscreen ✓
  (Behind & Inside Ear!)
- Meditate: Be Here Now! ✓
- Exercise: Walk & Swim ✓
- Eat Whole Foods ✓
- Take Vitamins & Pills ✓
- Call Loved Ones ✓
- Don't Talk About Yesterday – Only Today and Tomorrow ✓
- Don't Talk About Daily Bad News of Doom and Gloom ✓
- Open New Chapter
  Pursue a Passion ✓
- Epson Salt Bath ✓
  (Soothes Sore Muscles)
- Catch a FL Sunset ✓
- After Every Rain,
  Catch a FL Rainbow! ✓

Shift 5. 6-9 P.M.

Shift 6. 9-Midnight

Shift 7. Night Owl: 1-3 A.M.

Never regret a day in your life:
Good days give happiness.
Bad days give experience.
Worst days give lessons.
Dr. Sukhraj Dhillon

DO, DOING (DIY or Delegate), and DONE

Practice Daily Gratitude

I am grateful for: ______________________________

Practice: "Mindfulness, Meditation, and Mantra Mitigates Madness" S. Lampert
Mantra: ______________________________

Healthy Food Choices: Watch Your Weight!

Breakfast: ____________________

Lunch: ____________________

Dinner: ____________________

Snacks: ____________________

Exercise:
Walk, Gym, Tennis, Golf, Swim

____________________❑Done

Daily Tasks: DIY or Delegate?

____________________❑Done

____________________❑Done

____________________❑Done

Set Up Restaurant Reservations:

____________________❑Done

Phone Calls: Family and Social Life

____________________❑Done

____________________❑Done

Phone Calls: Business

____________________❑Done

____________________❑Done

Set Up Doctor Appointments:

____________________❑Done

____________________❑Done

Free Time—Me Time

Read Book: ____________________

Watch Movie: ____________________

TV Show: ____________________

Travel: ____________________

Night Life: ____________________

Random Acts of Kindness:

____________________❑Done

____________________❑Done

Household Chores:

____________________❑Done

____________________❑Done

Run Errands:

____________________❑Done

____________________❑Done

Buy Stuff or Groceries:

____________________❑Done

____________________❑Done

____________________❑Done

____________________❑Done

The perfect time to start something never arrives

START NOW!

7 Shifts: Time Management

Date: _______________

Shift 1. Early Bird: 5-8 A.M.

Shift 2. 9-Noon

Shift 3. Noon-3 P.M.

Shift 4. 3-6 P.M.

My Daily Routine:

- Catch a FL Sunrise ✓
- Check Your POOP! ✓
  Are You Hydrated? ✓
- Bag Pet POOP! ✓
- Appy Sunscreen ✓
  (Behind & Inside Ear!)
- Meditate: Be Here Now! ✓
- Exercise: Walk & Swim ✓
- Eat Whole Foods ✓
- Take Vitamins & Pills ✓
- Call Loved Ones ✓
- Don't Talk About Yesterday – Only Today and Tomorrow ✓
- Don't Talk About Daily Bad News of Doom and Gloom ✓
- Open New Chapter
  Pursue a Passion ✓
- Epson Salt Bath ✓
  (Soothes Sore Muscles)
- Catch a FL Sunset ✓
- After Every Rain, Catch a FL Rainbow! ✓

Shift 5. 6-9 P.M.

Shift 6. 9-Midnight

Shift 7. Night Owl: 1-3 A.M.

Never regret a day in your life:
Good days give happiness.
Bad days give experience.
Worst days give lessons.
Dr. Sukhraj Dhillon

DO, DOING (DIY or Delegate), and DONE

Practice Daily Gratitude

I am grateful for: ____________________

Practice: "Mindfulness, Meditation, and Mantra Mitigates Madness" S. Lampert
Mantra: ____________________

Healthy Food Choices: Watch Your Weight!

Breakfast: ____________________

Lunch: ____________________

Dinner: ____________________

Snacks: ____________________

Exercise:
Walk, Gym, Tennis, Golf, Swim

____________________ ❑Done

Daily Tasks: DIY or Delegate?

____________________ ❑Done

____________________ ❑Done

____________________ ❑Done

Set Up Restaurant Reservations:

____________________ ❑Done

Phone Calls: Family and Social Life

____________________ ❑Done

____________________ ❑Done

Phone Calls: Business

____________________ ❑Done

____________________ ❑Done

Set Up Doctor Appointments:

____________________ ❑Done

____________________ ❑Done

Free Time—Me Time

Read Book: ____________________

Watch Movie: ____________________

TV Show: ____________________

Travel: ____________________

Night Life: ____________________

Random Acts of Kindness:

____________________ ❑Done

____________________ ❑Done

Household Chores:

____________________ ❑Done

____________________ ❑Done

Run Errands:

____________________ ❑Done

____________________ ❑Done

Buy Stuff or Groceries:

____________________ ❑Done

____________________ ❑Done

____________________ ❑Done

____________________ ❑Done

The perfect time to start something never arrives

START NOW!

7 Shifts: Time Management

Date: ________________

Shift 1. Early Bird: 5-8 A.M.

Shift 2. 9-Noon

Shift 3. Noon-3 P.M.

Shift 4. 3-6 P.M.

My Daily Routine:

- Catch a FL Sunrise ✓
- Check Your POOP! ✓
  Are You Hydrated? ✓
- Bag Pet POOP! ✓
- Appy Sunscreen ✓
  (Behind & Inside Ear!)
- Meditate: Be Here Now! ✓
- Exercise: Walk & Swim ✓
- Eat Whole Foods ✓
- Take Vitamins & Pills ✓
- Call Loved Ones ✓
- Don't Talk About
  Yesterday – Only
  Today and Tomorrow ✓
- Don't Talk About
  Daily Bad News of
  Doom and Gloom ✓
- Open New Chapter
  Pursue a Passion ✓
- Epson Salt Bath ✓
  (Soothes Sore Muscles)
- Catch a FL Sunset ✓
- After Every Rain,
  Catch a FL Rainbow! ✓

Shift 5. 6-9 P.M.

Shift 6. 9-Midnight

Shift 7. Night Owl: 1-3 A.M.

Never regret a day in your life:
Good days give happiness.
Bad days give experience.
Worst days give lessons.
Dr. Sukhraj Dhillon

DO, DOING (DIY or Delegate), and DONE

Practice Daily Gratitude

I am grateful for: ______________________________

Practice: "Mindfulness, Meditation, and Mantra Mitigates Madness" S. Lampert
Mantra: ______________________________

Healthy Food Choices: Watch Your Weight!

Breakfast: ____________________

Lunch: ____________________

Dinner: ____________________

Snacks: ____________________

Exercise:
Walk, Gym, Tennis, Golf, Swim

____________________ ❑Done

Daily Tasks: DIY or Delegate?

____________________ ❑Done

____________________ ❑Done

____________________ ❑Done

Set Up Restaurant Reservations:

____________________ ❑Done

Phone Calls: Family and Social Life

____________________ ❑Done

____________________ ❑Done

Phone Calls: Business

____________________ ❑Done

____________________ ❑Done

Set Up Doctor Appointments:

____________________ ❑Done

____________________ ❑Done

Free Time—Me Time

Read Book: ____________________

Watch Movie: ____________________

TV Show: ____________________

Travel: ____________________

Night Life: ____________________

Random Acts of Kindness:

____________________ ❑Done

____________________ ❑Done

Household Chores:

____________________ ❑Done

____________________ ❑Done

Run Errands:

____________________ ❑Done

____________________ ❑Done

Buy Stuff or Groceries:

____________________ ❑Done

____________________ ❑Done

____________________ ❑Done

____________________ ❑Done

The perfect time to start something never arrives

START NOW!

7 Shifts: Time Management

Date: ________________

Shift 1. Early Bird: 5-8 A.M.

Shift 2. 9-Noon

Shift 3. Noon-3 P.M.

Shift 4. 3-6 P.M.

My Daily Routine:

- Catch a FL Sunrise ✓
- Check Your POOP! ✓
  Are You Hydrated? ✓
- Bag Pet POOP! ✓
- Appy Sunscreen ✓
  (Behind & Inside Ear!)
- Meditate: Be Here Now! ✓
- Exercise: Walk & Swim ✓
- Eat Whole Foods ✓
- Take Vitamins & Pills ✓
- Call Loved Ones ✓
- Don't Talk About Yesterday – Only Today and Tomorrow ✓
- Don't Talk About Daily Bad News of Doom and Gloom ✓
- Open New Chapter
  Pursue a Passion ✓
- Epson Salt Bath ✓
  (Soothes Sore Muscles)
- Catch a FL Sunset ✓
- After Every Rain, Catch a FL Rainbow! ✓

Shift 5. 6-9 P.M.

Shift 6. 9-Midnight

Shift 7. Night Owl: 1-3 A.M.

Never regret a day in your life:
Good days give happiness.
Bad days give experience.
Worst days give lessons.
Dr. Sukhraj Dhillon

The Facts of Aging

by Mimi Gould (Atlanta, Georgia)

So much to do before I pass
and here I sit upon my ass,
my energy is gone there's none to spare
I lay on the bed, still in my underwear.

I wasn't warned about getting old
I tried to do what I was told
but none advised me about fatigue,
and laziness and the lack of speed.

I munch on ice cream and candy bars
and wonder how my waist got large.
I truly want an exercise routine
but end up with People magazine.

It's disgusting to me, this aging event,
I can't even remember how my days are spent.
The golden years are simply phony
with time to spare, it's pure baloney!

I'll wake up tomorrow and hear myself say,
hooray, I'm vertical for another day.
And suddenly the day goes by,
hours seem like seconds, the time just flies.

The months and years are gone like a breeze.
I need more days, dear GOD, if you please.
A new year is here, I must take control
of mind and body and this lazy soul.

I'll rid the cupboards of cookies and sweets
and try my darndest to get off my seat.
The stationery bike awaits my butt,
and perhaps a dance class to strut my stuff.

I've letters to write and a canvas to paint on
and a memoir to write before I'm gone.
I used to run just like a bunny,
batteries charged, yes, that was me.

Now I'm down to a turtle pace,
the only speed are wrinkles on my face.
Dear GOD, please hear my prayer,
bless me with vigor and enough to share.

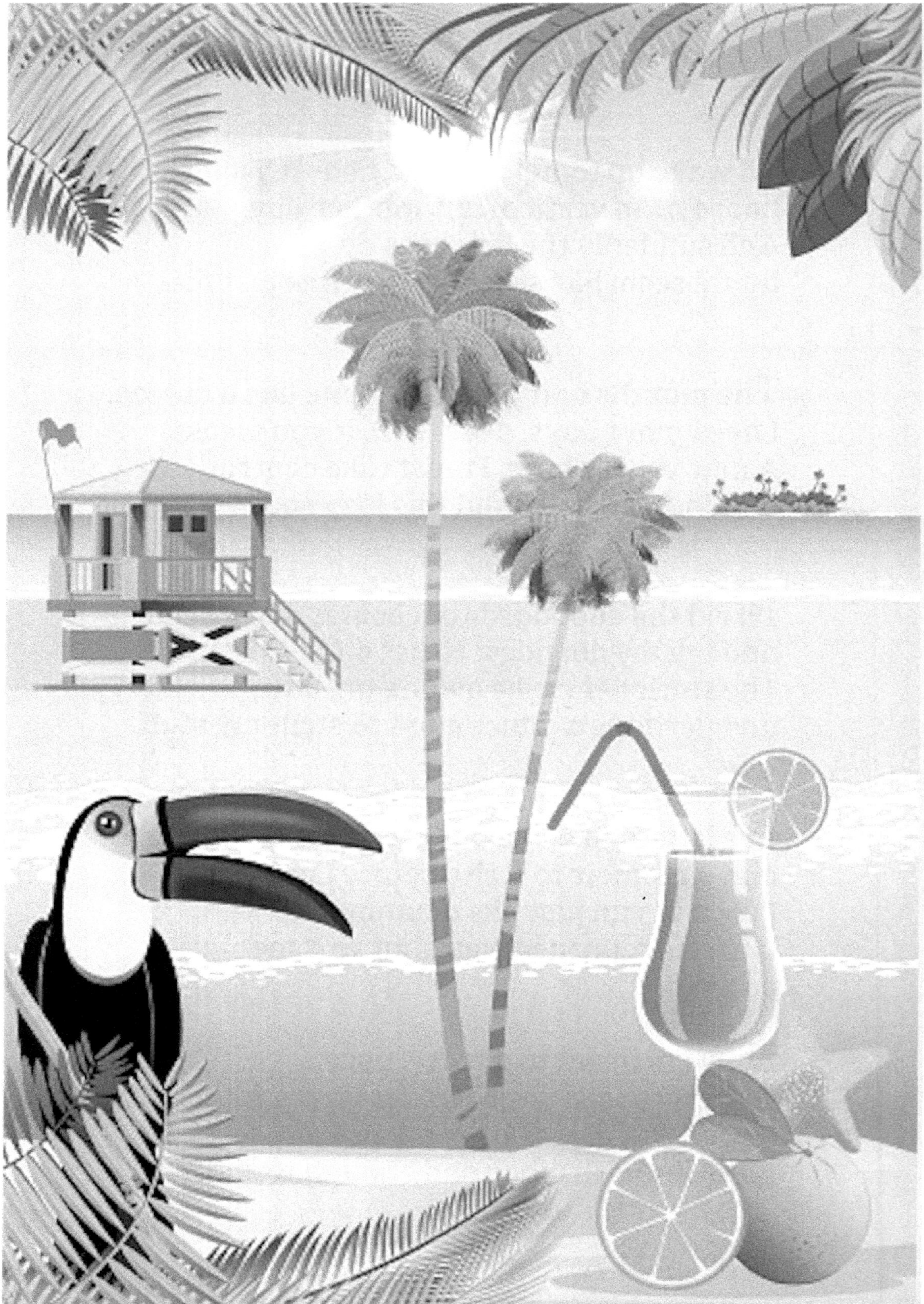

My Travel Log, Note Pad, and Journal

Write Down Your Family History

Write it All Down Before You Forget to Pass on the Information to the Next Generation

My Travel Log, Notepad, and Journal

My Travel Log, Notepad, and Journal

My Travel Log, Notepad, and Journal

My Travel Log, Notepad, and Journal

My Travel Log, Notepad, and Journal

My Travel Log, Notepad, and Journal

My Travel Log, Notepad, and Journal

My Travel Log, Notepad, and Journal

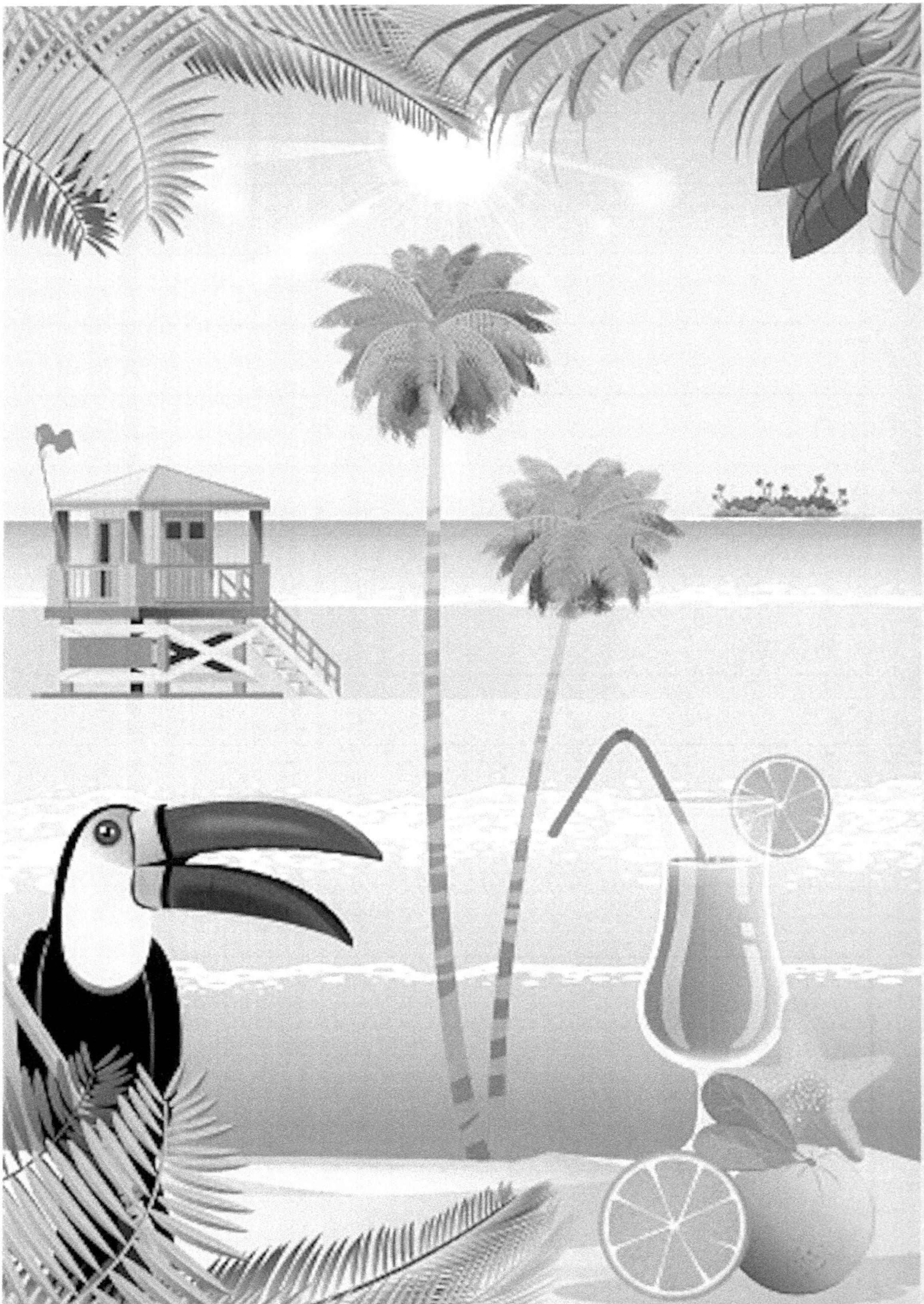

My Organizer

Retirement: 5-Year Life Transitions p.52
Mental Health pp.53-55
Healthy Food Choices p.56
Lose Weight and Keep the Weight Off p.57
Computer Passwords pp.58-59
Doctors & Daily Medications pp.60-61

Family Reminders:

Birthday Reminders pp.62-63
Beloved Grandchildren and the Adorble
Things Grandkids Say and Do! pp.64-65
Important Phone Numbers pp.66-67

Legal Reminders:

Lawyer, Accountant, Financial Advisor and,
Banking Information pp.68-69

Free Time—Me Time

6 Survival Dating Tips p.71
Favorite Books & Movies pp.72-73
11 Golf Pro Tips pp.74-75
7 Tennis Pro Tips pp.76-77
28 Games: Card, Board, Group, and Solo pp.78-79
Join the Digital Revolution pp.80-81

Retirement: 5-Year Life Transitions

Now that you have retired, you are busier than ever before – how can you fit it all in during retirement? Life changes every 5 years, and now is the right time to start planning for your next set of life transitions:

Transition 1: Ages 65-70
- Stay active, so that you have something to talk about — or you will only talk about yesterday, when you had a life!
- You are free to be a night owl and sleep late until noon.
- You will have to rethink your social life, and the dating world.
- If you have an active night life, you may need an afternoon nap.

Transition 2: Ages 70-75
- Most of your peers have a medical condition, and are on medication.
- No dating breakups any more – couples change partners when the partner passes away. Women change boyfriends every decade.
- Every other senior has skin cancer and needs Mohs surgery! (SUNSCREEN)

Transition 3: Ages 75-80
- You kids start treating you like an extra set of kids, and ask you to call them once a day, to tell them everything. Find something to talk about besides the doctor, diagnosis, disease, dying, and death.
- "Who died today?" is the main topic of conversation.
- Aging is about "loss." What did you lose today?

Transition 4: Ages 80-85
- You will probably start taking afternoon naps each day.
- The less you remember from the past, the less aggravation you feel.
- Men who are alive past age 80 have plenty of women fighting over them!
- Your peers are dying, and you will have to learn how to make new friends.

Transition 5: Ages 85-90
- You will need to rethink your ability to drive a car safely.
- You will need to be aware of the signs of dementia/Alzheimer's.
- First sign of dementia: You don't remember where you put your things, and accuse people of stealing your stuff.
- Most of your peers are dead and buried, and your new friends are younger.

Transition 6: Ages 90-95
- You may outlive your own children.
- You flirt with the nurse and this behavior is adorable— not offensive.
- You move into an assisted living facility.
- You listen to audio books mailed directed to your home: Library for the Blind.

Transition 7: Ages 95-100
- Lucky you! The newspapers will celebrate you with a feature article: 100!

My Mental Health

• My Daily Gratitude Workout

• My Positive Thinking Workout

Florida is "God's Waiting Room"
Retirement is the first chapter
before life's final chapters:
• Nursing Home
• Hospice
• Cemetery
Life moves fast, and is fragile and finite.

Retirement is either a blessing or a curse?
You can fulfill a lifelong PASSION like
writing a book or traveling the world,
or spend it visiting doctors' offices, and
calling your kids daily to discuss the 9 "D"
words as you fight for an extension of life!
1. Daily
2. Discussion
3&4. Daughter Donna ________________
5. Doctor
6. Diagnosis
7. Disease
8. Dying
9. Death

My Gratitude Workout

I Am Grateful for All the Blessings in My Life

1. I am grateful for: ______________________________
2. I am grateful for: ______________________________
3. I am grateful for: ______________________________
4. I am grateful for: ______________________________
5. I am grateful for: ______________________________
6. I am grateful for: ______________________________
7. I am grateful for: ______________________________

Count Your Blessings

Count your blessings instead of your crosses;
Count your gains instead of your losses.

Count your joys instead of your woes;
Count your friends instead of your foes.

Count your smiles instead of your tears;
Count your courage instead of your fears.

Count your full years instead of your lean;
Count your kind deeds instead of your mean.

Count your health instead of your wealth;
Love your neighbor as much as yourself.

My Positive Affirmation Workout

Don't Ruin a Good Today
Thinking About a Bad Yesterday!

Unknown

Good People, Nothing Is a Problem!
Bad People, Everything Is a Problem!

Sharon Esther Lampert

All People Help You with Their Strengths
And Hurt You With Their Weaknesses

Sharon Esther Lampert

All You Get for Negativity Is
NOTHING

Sharon Esther Lampert

A UNIVERSAL MORAL COMPASS

FOR ALL PEOPLE, FOR ALL RELIGIONS, FOR ALL TIME

The 22 Commandments by Philosopher Queen Sharon Esther Lampert

1. **LIFE** Over Death
2. **STRENGTH** Over Weakness
3. **DEED** Over Sin
4. **LOVE** Over Hatred
5. **TRUTH** Over Lie
6. **COURAGE** Over Fear
7. **OPTIMISM** Over Pessimism
8. **SHARING** Over Selfishness
9. **PRAISE** Over Criticism
10. **LOYALTY** Over Abandonment
11. **RESPONSIBILITY** Over Blame
12. **GRATITUDE** Over Envy
13. **REWARD** Over Punishment
14. **GENEROUS** Over Stingy
15. **CREATION** Over Destruction
16. **EDUCATION** Over Ignorance
17. **COOPERATION** Over Competition
18. **FREEDOM** Over Oppression
19. **COMPASSION** Over Indifference
20. **FORGIVENESS** Over Revenge
21. **PEACE** Over War
22. **JOY** Over Suffering

My Grocery List of Healthy Food Choices

1. ______________________________
2. ______________________________
3. ______________________________
.
4. ______________________________
5. ______________________________
6. ______________________________
7. ______________________________
8. ______________________________
9. ______________________________
10. ______________________________
11. ______________________________
12. ______________________________
13. ______________________________
14. ______________________________
15. ______________________________
16. ______________________________
17. ______________________________
18. ______________________________

Reminders:

1. Choose whole foods over processed food, junk food, and fast food ✓
2. Whole foods do not need an ingredient label ✓
3. Eat Smaller Portions ✓
   Eat Slowly ✓
   Don't Gobble ✓
4. Avoid addictive foods loaded with salt and sugar ✓
5. Chemicals cause inflammation and disease ✓
6. When eating out, cut portion in half, and take home ✓
7. When eating out, pick baked over fried foods✓
8. Freeze Food for Zero Waste ✓
9. Food Is Medicine and Fuel:
   ✓Good Protein vs. Bad Protein
   ✓Good Fats vs. Bad Fats
   ✓Good Carbs vs. Bad Carbs

Lose Weight and Keep the Weight Off

1. Never leave the condo on an empty stomach. Filler up! Always pack a sandwich bag with an apple, carrot and celery sticks, and a bottle of water. Stay hydrated!

2. Plan your meals in advance. You will no longer be tempted to eat the wrong foods, because you are never looking for something to eat —a bad habit— that will end with you putting on extra pounds: fast food, junk food, and processed food. Eat a plant based nutrient-dense diet.

   Breakfast: Green Drink: Watermelon, Mint, Parsely
   Lunch: Mixed Vegetables and a Protein (Meat/Fish)
   Dinner: Broccoli, Sardines and Crumbled Goat Cheese

3. As soon as your meal is served, cut it in half, and ask for a doggy bag, and bring it home. Restaurant platters are for 2-3 people. Stop eating food for two or three people!

4. If you don't want to walk around with a doggy bag— restaurants serve a bowl of soup and half a sandwich. This is a great option to maintain a slim waistline.

5. Sharing one entree with a friend is an excellent option for eating a smaller perfect portion of food, and not walking around with a doggy bag.

6. If I asked you to eat a three cups of sugar and a stick of butter—you would adamantly decline the request. Every cake or cookie is made of three cups of sugar and a stick of butter. Zero nutrition and extra pounds are the price you pay for a sweet tooth! Apples come in 20 different variaties, and are packed with nutrition, crunch, and long-lasting energy in the form of fiber.

My Computer Passwords

Date: ___________
Website: __________________________
Email/User Name: ______________________
Password: ______________________

Date: ___________
Website: __________________________
Email/User Name: ______________________
Password: ______________________

Date: ___________
Website: __________________________
Email/User Name: ______________________
Password: ______________________

Date: ___________
Website: __________________________
Email/User Name: ______________________
Password: ______________________

Date: ___________
Website: __________________________
Email/User Name: ______________________
Password: ______________________

Date: ___________
Website: __________________________
Email/User Name: ______________________
Password: ______________________

My Computer Passwords

Date: __________
Website: ________________________
Email/User Name: ____________________
Password: ____________________

Date: __________
Website: ________________________
Email/User Name: ____________________
Password: ____________________

Date: __________
Website: ________________________
Email/User Name: ____________________
Password: ____________________

Date: __________
Website: ________________________
Email/User Name: ____________________
Password: ____________________

Date: __________
Website: ________________________
Email/User Name: ____________________
Password: ____________________

Date: __________
Website: ________________________
Email/User Name: ____________________
Password: ____________________

My Doctors & Daily Medications

Doctor's Name: ______________________________
Office Assistant's Name: ______________________________
Address: ______________________________
Office Phone# ______________________________
Emergency# ______________________________
Office Email: ______________________________
Medications: ______________________________
How Many Times a Day? ______________________________
What Time During the Day? ______________________________
Notes: ______________________________
____

Doctor's Name: ______________________________
Office Assistant's Name: ______________________________
Address: ______________________________
Office Phone# ______________________________
Emergency# ______________________________
Office Email: ______________________________
Medications: ______________________________
How Many Times a Day? ______________________________
What Time During the Day? ______________________________
Notes: ______________________________
____

Doctor's Name: ______________________________
Office Assistant's Name: ______________________________
Address: ______________________________
Office Phone# ______________________________
Emergency# ______________________________
Office Email: ______________________________
Medications: ______________________________
How Many Times a Day? ______________________________
What Time During the Day? ______________________________
Notes: ______________________________
____

My Doctors & Daily Medications

Doctor's Name: ______________________________
Office Assistant's Name: ______________________________
Address: ______________________________
Office Phone# ______________________________
Emergency# ______________________________
Office Email: ______________________________
Medications: ______________________________
How Many Times a Day? ______________________________
What Time During the Day? ______________________________
Notes: ______________________________
____

Doctor's Name: ______________________________
Office Assistant's Name: ______________________________
Address: ______________________________
Office Phone# ______________________________
Emergency# ______________________________
Office Email: ______________________________
Medications: ______________________________
How Many Times a Day? ______________________________
What Time During the Day? ______________________________
Notes: ______________________________
____

Doctor's Name: ______________________________
Office Assistant's Name: ______________________________
Address: ______________________________
Office Phone# ______________________________
Emergency# ______________________________
Office Email: ______________________________
Medications: ______________________________
How Many Times a Day? ______________________________
What Time During the Day? ______________________________
Notes: ______________________________
____

My Birthday Reminders

Name: ______________________________
Birthday: ______________________________
Gift Ideas: ______________________________
Phone Number: ______________________________

Name: ______________________________
Birthday: ______________________________
Gift Ideas: ______________________________
Phone Number: ______________________________

Name: ______________________________
Birthday: ______________________________
Gift Ideas: ______________________________
Phone Number: ______________________________

Name: ______________________________
Birthday: ______________________________
Gift Ideas: ______________________________
Phone Number: ______________________________

Name: ______________________________
Birthday: ______________________________
Gift Ideas: ______________________________
Phone Number: ______________________________

Name: ______________________________
Birthday: ______________________________
Gift Ideas: ______________________________
Phone Number: ______________________________

Name: ______________________________
Birthday: ______________________________
Gift Ideas: ______________________________

My Birthday Reminders

Name: ______________________________
Birthday: ______________________________
Gift Ideas: ______________________________
Phone Number: ______________________________

Name: ______________________________
Birthday: ______________________________
Gift Ideas: ______________________________
Phone Number: ______________________________

Name: ______________________________
Birthday: ______________________________
Gift Ideas: ______________________________
Phone Number: ______________________________

Name: ______________________________
Birthday: ______________________________
Gift Ideas: ______________________________
Phone Number: ______________________________

Name: ______________________________
Birthday: ______________________________
Gift Ideas: ______________________________
Phone Number: ______________________________

Name: ______________________________
Birthday: ______________________________
Gift Ideas: ______________________________
Phone Number: ______________________________

Name: ______________________________
Birthday: ______________________________
Gift Ideas: ______________________________

My Beloved Grandchildren

Grandchild's Full Name: ____________________
Named After: ____________________
Nickname: ____________________
Birthday: ____________________
Favorite Foods: ____________________
Favorite Books: ____________________
Favorite Music: ____________________
Likes: ____________________
Dislikes: ____________________

Adorable Things My Grandchild Says and Does

____
____
____

Grandchild's Full Name: ____________________
Named After: ____________________
Nickname: ____________________
Birthday: ____________________
Favorite Foods: ____________________
Favorite Books: ____________________
Favorite Music: ____________________
Likes: ____________________
Dislikes: ____________________

Adorable Things My Grandchild Says and Does

____
____
____

My Beloved Grandchildren

Grandchild's Full Name: ____________________
Named After: ____________________
Nickname: ____________________
Birthday: ____________________
Favorite Foods: ____________________
Favorite Books: ____________________
Favorite Music: ____________________
Likes: ____________________
Dislikes: ____________________

Adorable Things My Grandchild Says and Does

____
____
____

Grandchild's Full Name: ____________________
Named After: ____________________
Nickname: ____________________
Birthday: ____________________
Favorite Foods: ____________________
Favorite Books: ____________________
Favorite Music: ____________________
Likes: ____________________
Dislikes: ____________________

Adorable Things My Grandchild Says and Does

____
____
____

Important Phone Numbers

Name: ______________________________
Address: ______________________________
Phone: ______________________________
Cell Phone: ______________________________
Email: ______________________________
Website: ______________________________
Notes: ______________________________

Name: ______________________________
Address: ______________________________
Phone: ______________________________
Cell Phone: ______________________________
Email: ______________________________
Website: ______________________________
Notes: ______________________________

Name: ______________________________
Address: ______________________________
Phone: ______________________________
Cell Phone: ______________________________
Email: ______________________________
Website: ______________________________
Notes: ______________________________

Name: ______________________________
Address: ______________________________
Phone: ______________________________
Cell Phone: ______________________________
Email: ______________________________
Website: ______________________________
Notes: ______________________________

Important Phone Numbers

Name: ______________________________
Address: ______________________________
Phone: ______________________________
Cell Phone: ______________________________
Email: ______________________________
Website: ______________________________
Notes: ______________________________

Name: ______________________________
Address: ______________________________
Phone: ______________________________
Cell Phone: ______________________________
Email: ______________________________
Website: ______________________________
Notes: ______________________________

Name: ______________________________
Address: ______________________________
Phone: ______________________________
Cell Phone: ______________________________
Email: ______________________________
Website: ______________________________
Notes: ______________________________

Name: ______________________________
Address: ______________________________
Phone: ______________________________
Cell Phone: ______________________________
Email: ______________________________
Website: ______________________________
Notes: ______________________________

My Lawyer, Account, and Financial Advisors

Lawyer

Company Name: ______________________________
Name: ______________________________
Office Assistant's Name: ______________________________
Office Phone: ______________________________
Address: ______________________________
Email: ______________________________

1. Will 2. Power of Attorney 3. Medical Directive 4. Trusts

Accountant

Company Name: ______________________________
Name: ______________________________
Office Assistant's Name: ______________________________
Office Phone: ______________________________
Address: ______________________________
Email: ______________________________

Financial Advisor

Company Name: ______________________________
Name: ______________________________
Office Assistant's Name: ______________________________
Office Phone: ______________________________
Address: ______________________________
Email: ______________________________

My Banking Information

Bank Name: ____________________
Account #: ____________________
Banker's Name: ____________________
Bank Phone#: ____________________
Address: ____________________
Banker's Email: ____________________

Bank Name: ____________________
Account #: ____________________
Banker's Name: ____________________
Bank Phone#: ____________________
Address: ____________________
Banker's Email: ____________________

Bank Name: ____________________
Account #: ____________________
Banker's Name: ____________________
Bank Phone#: ____________________
Address: ____________________
Banker's Email: ____________________

Bank Name: ____________________
Account #: ____________________
Banker's Name: ____________________
Bank Phone#: ____________________
Address: ____________________
Banker's Email: ____________________

Bank Name: ____________________
Account #: ____________________
Banker's Name: ____________________
Bank Phone#: ____________________
Address: ____________________

Free Time–Me Time

- 6 Dating Survival Tips
- Great Books
- Great Movies
- 11 Pro Golf Tips
- 7 Tennis Pro Tips
- 28 Card Games
- Social Media
- Passion Project: Write a Book

6 Dating Survival Tips

1. Everyone you meet is on a different dating plan, so best to ask the simple but profound question: "What dating plan are you on?"
Plan A. Marriage
Plan B. Monogamous Boyfriend - Girlfriend Relationship
Plan C. Dating Many Different People at the Same Time
Plan D. One-Night Stand

2. **Dating Safety:** When setting up a first, second, and third date, meet in a public place, and drive yourself home. Let a friend know where you will be. Keep a diary of RED FLAGS!

3. **Avoid Oversharing:** Keep the conversation light – no religion, politics, and painful life experiences. Leave yesterday behind! Talk about today and tomorrow. Make them laugh—not cry!

4. **Get Tested!:** Sexually transmitted diseases are the highest among seniors because many sexually active seniors forgo protection when they have a sexual encounter. It's important to protect yourself. To keep you and your partner safe, get tested at least once a year, and use condoms if you are unsure of your partner's sexual history.

5. **One True Love Every Decade:** Women change partners every decade—there are no more breakups or divorce—because the men usually die first.
Age 60: Husband: Divorce or Death
Age 70: New Boyfriend (and in-between Love Affairs)
Age 80: New Boyfriend (and in-between Love Affairs)
Age: 90: New and Last True Love!
Take note: Men who are alive past age 80 have hundreds of girlfriends!

6. **Privacy:** Suitors will check out your social-media accounts first—so don't post your really personal love life. Maintain your privacy!

Favorite Books or Recommendations

Title: ____

Author: ____

Title: ____

Author: ____

Title: ____

Author: ____

Title: ____

Author: ____

Title: ____

Author: ____

Title: ____

Author: ____

Title: ____

Author: ____

Title: ____

Author: ____

Favorite Movies or Recommendations

Movie: ______________________________

Movie: ______________________________

Movie: ______________________________

Movie: ______________________________

Movie: ______________________________

Movie: ______________________________

Movie: ______________________________

Movie: ______________________________

Movie: ______________________________

Movie: ______________________________

Movie: ______________________________

Movie: ______________________________

Movie: ______________________________

My 11 Golf Pro Tips

1. **Swing with an Anti-Slice Grip**
To improve your ability to deliver a square clubface (relative to your path), make practice swings with your hands split apart on the grip.

2. **3 Steps to Perfect Posture**
To correctly prep your posture for action, stand with a club pressed against your thighs.

3. **Get Square at the Start**
Place an alignment stick just outside the golf ball, so it creates a 90-degree angle with the target line.

4. **Check your Putter Path:** Use a straight or arcing stroke.

5. **Get Wide Early for Speed Where It Counts**
In order to create maximum speed, you have to create maximum width.

6. **One Drill for Better Driving:** Extend arms fully through impact.

7. **Whip Up More Speed**
"Snap" your wrists and hands through the strike without over swinging your shoulders.

8. **Stop Chips on a Dime**
Hit down on the ball sharply and with lots of acceleration — two keys for creating max short-game spin.

9. **Square up Your Stance from the Bunker**
Dig the blade into the sand to gouge the ball out, as if you're playing from a buried lie.

10. **Learn to Keep Your Head Still in Your Swing**

11. **The Right Way to Take a Speed Grip**
Set grip diagonally across your digits, and then wrap your thumb pad over the top of the handle. Pour on the speed!

My Golf Score Card (pencil)

Holes	Par	Score
Hole 1		
Hole 2		
Hole 3		
Hole 4		
Hole 5		
Hole 6		
Hole 7		
Hole 8		
Hole 9		

Friend: ______________________

Holes	Par	Score
Hole 1		
Hole 2		
Hole 3		
Hole 4		
Hole 5		
Hole 6		
Hole 7		
Hole 8		
Hole 9		

My 7 Tennis Pro Tips

1. **Early Preparation**
   GET THAT RACQUET BACK!
   You cannot prepare soon enough! Turn your hips and shoulders before the oncoming ball bounces on your side.

2. **Exaggerate Your Follow Through**
   MOVE YOUR FEET!
   Exaggerate your follow-through; do not think, just hit the ball.

3. **Two Bounces and You're Out**
   DON'T THINK, JUST RUN FOR THE BALL!
   Whenever you rally, wherever you play, make up your mind that you will never let the ball bounce twice. Always run for the ball even if you think you have no chance to reach it. Whatever comes to you, it is in play!

4. **Hit-Recover**
   Just Hit, Finish and Get Back to Position!
   So many players will hit a ball and watch the ball and compliment themselves on the shot. From now on you must hit and recover. Pros are recovering in the middle of their hit.

5. **Foundation Warm-Ups**
   Start at the serve line but stand in between the singles and doubles lines. Rally or play points hitting only between the lines. As you gain confidence, move back farther until you are on the baseline.

6. **A Safety Target**
   Build Points on Offense
   Players overplay the ball, including playing the lines. Watch how the pros build points, they play offensive but do not go for just winners.

7. **Practice Warm-Up Serves Before Serving**
   Get into serve position; practice first serve, hit second serve.

My Tennis Score

0 points = Love
1 point = 15
2 points = 30
3 points = 40
Tied score = All
40-40 = Deuce

Game, Set, and Match

SET: is collection of games, played until a player wins six games (or more).

MATCH: is played to a best-of-three or five sets. Championship matches are played to five sets.

	Set 1	Set 2	Set 3
Player A	6	5	6
Player B	4	7	1

Tennis Scoring Rules

There are multiple ways a point can be scored. Among them:

- An unreturnable ball (ball bounces twice) Double fault;
- Ace (unreturnable serve)
- Ball hit out of bounds (the lines count as in)
- Ball hit into the net

28 Games: Card, Board, Groups, and Solo

Thousands of retired seniors play card games in social halls that are strictly dedicated to card games. The easiest way to strike up a conversation and make friends is to spend 3-5 hours at a card table, and play a few rounds of cards or board games.

Soon after, you and your friends will be meeting up at the pool, taking in a movie, and going out for dinner every week.

Later on, you may even take a cruise, and travel the world together.

Best of all, you will have friends who enjoy seeing the brand-new photo of your adorable grandchildren.

8 Fun Card Games

1. **Pinochle** is a popular senior card game with many variations.
2. **Bridge** is another card game that will help to keep the mind sharp.
3. **Canasta** was popular in the 1950s, making it a hit among today's seniors.
4. **Rummy** is a popular game worldwide, and is good for two to four players.
5. **Cribbage** is so well liked, it even has a membership club.
6. **Chinese poker** is a fun variation with 13 cards organized into three poker-style hands.
7. **Big two** is a competitive card game that involves smart strategy and prudent play.
8. **Solitaire** is a lifelong favorite card game with numerous variations.

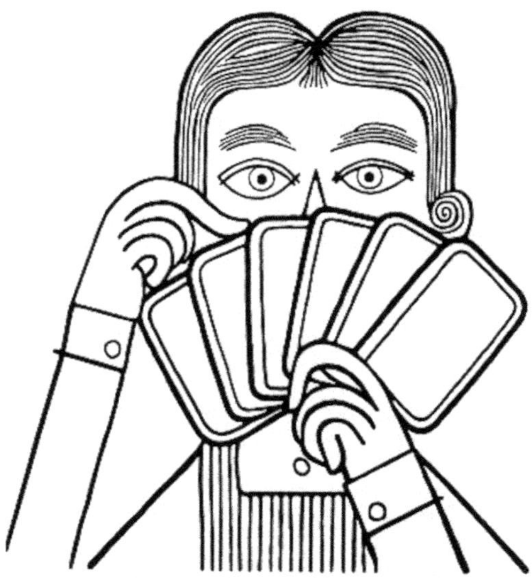

8 Fun Board Games

1. **Backgammon** is one of the oldest board games in the world.
2. **Scrabble** is a tiled word game that will challenge vocabulary skills.
3. **Go** is a board game of Asian origin and shares similarities with **Othello** and **Reversi.**
4. **Chess** challenges players to think several steps ahead of their opponents.
5. **Chinese checkers,** invented in Germany, is a great game for up to six players to enjoy.
6. **Trivial Pursuit** tests the knowledge and memory of players across six diverse categories.
7. **Hive** is a terrific abstract game that is easily played on any flat surface.

Fun Games to Play in Groups

1. **Mahjong** is a tile game for four players, vying to create the best possible hand to win.
2. **Bingo** is an old favorite that has always been popular with seniors and in casinos.
3. **Dominoes** is a tile-based game with numerous variations.
4. **Boggle** is a fast-paced word game that is more accessible than Scrabble.
5. **Yahtzee** is a simple dice game that borrows some elements from basic poker hands.
6. **Bocce** is a relaxing outdoor game that players of every fitness level can enjoy.
7. **Quoits** is a ring toss game that will elicit memories of visits to the local carnival.

Solo Puzzle Games

Puzzle games challenge the brain's problem-solving abilities, making them ideal for maintaining mental agility.

1. **Crossword puzzles** are normally played alone, testing vocabulary and expanding language skills.
2. **Sudoku** is a number-based puzzle game that appears regularly in newspapers.
3. **Match 3** games like **Candy Crush Saga** are available on PC, iPhone and Android.
4. **Jigsaw puzzles** are great to have around for seniors. You can start one on the coffee table or at a senior clubhouse, and work on it anytime.
5. **Word search** puzzles offer hours of fun.
6. **Word jumbles** can prove to be real brain teasers.

Join Digital Revolution

Email, Facebook, Twitter, and ZOOM

Part 1.
Set Up **Email** and Create **Password**

1. You need an email account to sign up for social media accounts. If you don't have an email account, you can set one up at **www.Gmail.com.**

2. You will also need a **PASSWORD**. Create a simple password that is easy to remember, Sample **PASSWORD**: pet's name followed by 1,2,3

   PASSWORD: mydogskip123

3. Use the same **EMAIL** and **PASSWORD** for all your social media accounts.

Part 2.
Set Up a **FACEBOOK** Account

Step 1. Open Facebook website and click on "Create an Account"
Go to **https://facebook.com/** in your computer's web browser.

Step 2. Enter your first name, your last name, a valid email address, your preferred password, your birthday, and then select whether you are male or female. Click **"Create an account"** when done.

Step 3. **Confirm your registration.** Facebook will send you a confirmation e-mail after signing up, so head the email address you used to sign up and click the confirmation e-mail.

Step 4. **Find friends.** Facebook will use your email contacts, and it will automatically send a friend request in your behalf.

Step 5. **Build your profile.** Enter your secondary school, college/university if applicable, employer, current city, and hometown.

Part 3.
Set Up a **TWITTER** Account

Step 1. Open Twitter website.
Go to **https://twitter.com/** in your computer's web browser.

Step 2. Click **Sign Up.** It's a blue button in the middle of the page.
This will take you to the Twitter sign-up page.

Step 3. Enter your name. Type your name into the "Name" text box.
The name you choose does not have to be your real name.

Step 4. Enter your email address.

Step 5. Click **Sign up.** This option is in the middle of the page.

Step 6. Enter your **PASSWORD**, then click Next to confirm your password.

Step 7. **Select interests.**
Scroll through the list of topics and click topics of interest.

Step 8. **Follow people.** Tap each account you want to follow.

Step 9. Complete Twitter set-up.

Part 4.

Set Up a **ZOOM** Account

Step 1. Navigate to https://www.zoom.us, enter your email address, and click on the **"Sign Up it's Free"** button.

Step 2. Verify that your address is correct and click **Confirm**.

Step 3. Click on the **"Activate Account"** button in the email message send to the account you specified.

Step 4. Continue the Zoom set-up by entering your name and selecting a **PASSWORD**. Please note the **password** requirements listed in red.

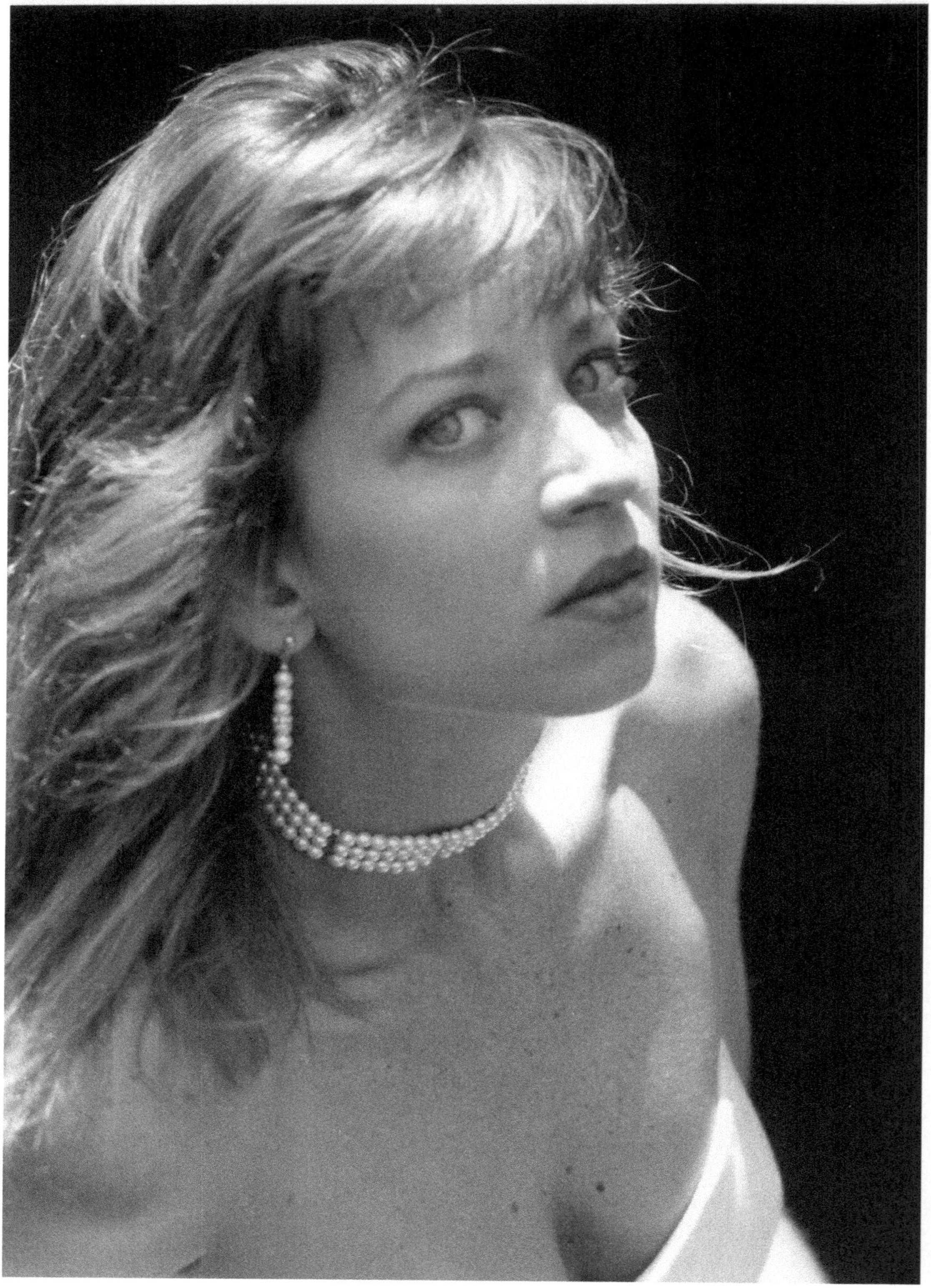

Sharon Esther Lampert

About the Author

SHARON ESTHER LAMPERT

V.E.S.S.E.L. Very. Extra. Special. Sharon. Esther. Lampert.

POET

The Greatest Poems Ever Written on Extraordinary World Events
(WorldFamousPoems.com, SharonEstherLampert.com, PoetryJewels.com)

PROPHET

GOD TALKS TO ME: A Working Definition of God
22 Commandments: All You Will Ever Need to Know About God
(PhilosopherQueen.com)

PHILOSOPHER

God of What: Is Life a Gift or a Punishment? 40 Absolute Truths
(GodofWhat.com)

PEACEMAKER

World Peace Equation
(WorldPeaceEquation.com)

PRODIGY

10 Esoteric Laws of Genius and Creativity
40 Rules of Manhood: For Men of All Ages
14 Relationship Strategies for Happily After Ever
13 Temporary Insanity—Written in the Letter S
CUPID Love Languages —Written in Letter C
My Day, My Dream, My Destiny—Written in Letter D
The Secret Sauce of Book Sales—Written in Letter P

PALADIN OF EDUCATION

40 Universal Gold Standards of Education
10 SMARTGRADES Tools to Ace Every Test Every Time
15 Stepping Stones of Academic Success
15 Stumbling Blocks of Academic Failure
www.Smartgrades.com

PHOTON

SUPERHERO OF EDUCATION
www.PhotonSuperhero.com

PIN-UP

PERFORMER

Vocalist: Ashira Orchestra (YouTube videos)

PLAYER: JOCK

NYU Women's Varsity Basketball Team

What is the #1 Topic of Conversation of Retired Seniors?

A. Travel: The Travel Addict
B. Books
C. Weight Loss
D. Money
E. Dating, Sex, and Love
F. Playing Cards
G. Grandchildren

A for Travel is the Correct Answer!

What is the #2 Topic of Conversation of Retired Seniors?

A. Travel
B. Books
C. Weight Loss: WIN AT THIN
D. Money
E. Dating, Sex, and Love
F. Playing Cards
G. Grandchildren

C for Health is the Correct Answer!

#2 Book of Retired Seniors Is:

WIN AT THIN
Fat Me, Skinny Me

www.SharonEstherLampert.com

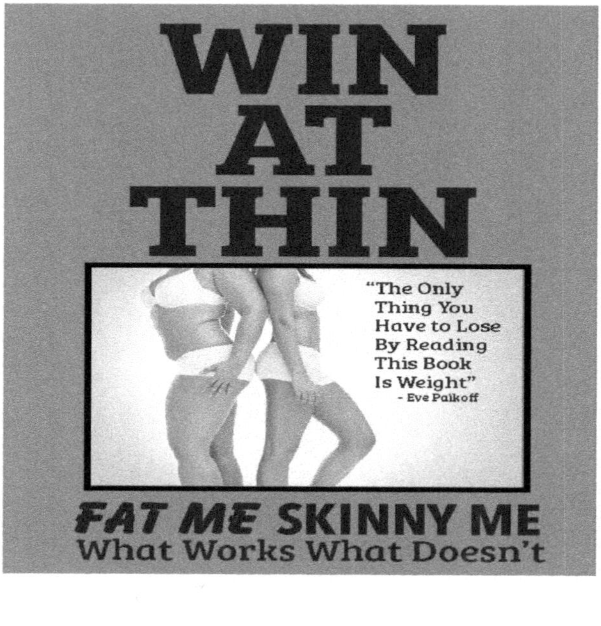

What is the #3 Topic of Conversation of Retired Seniors?

A. Travel
B. Life: The Miracle Memoir
C. Weight Loss
D. Money
E. Dating, Sex, and Love
F. Playing Cards
G. Grandchildren

B for Books is the Correct Answer!

#3 Book of Retired Seniors Is:

The Miracle Memoir

HURRAY I'M ALIVE!

Esther Tulkoff Is a Local Celebrity!

www.EstherTulkoff.com

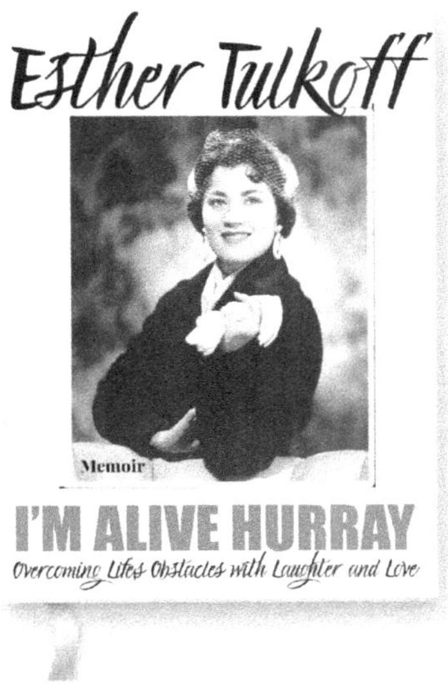

What is the #4 Topic of Conversation of Retired Seniors?

A. Travel
B. Books
C. Weight Loss
D. Money
E. Dating: SEX ON A PLATE
F. Playing Cards
G. Grandchildren

E for Dating is the Correct Answer!

#4 Book of Retired Seniors Is:

SEX ON A PLATE

Every Great Relationship Begins with the Perfect Meal

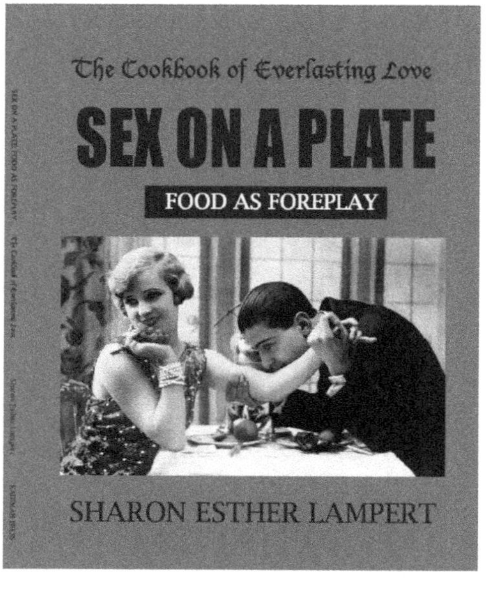

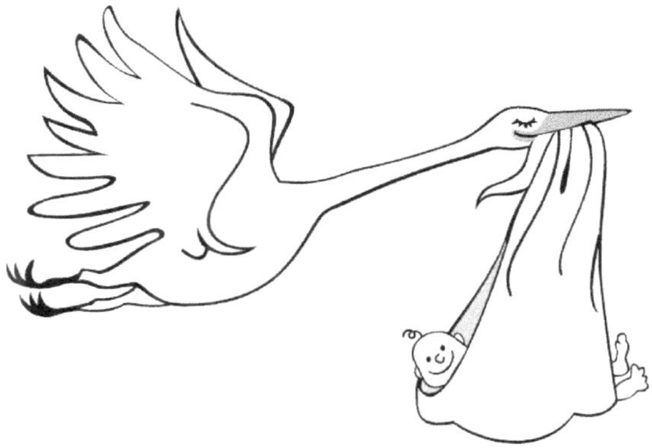

BE BORN

Become Educated.
Fulfill Your Potential.
Follow Your Passion.
Find Your Place in the World.
Make a Meaningful Contribution to
Your Family, Friends, and Humanity.
Self-Love Is True Love.
Be Your Own Best Friend.
Have Sex with Someone You Love.
Make Love with Complete Abandon.
Enjoy Unconditional Love from Your Devoted Pet.
Make Time to Read the Funnies and Laugh.
Save Enough Money to Visit the Popular, Pretty,
and Peaceful Places of the World.
Read Great Literature, Listen to Great Music
See Great Art, Watch the Great Movies
Play the Fun Sports, Dance Till Dawn
Taste the Great Culinary Delights of the World.
Eat Slowly, Enjoy Every Bite, and Stay in Shape.
Plan One Great Adventure and Stick to the Plan.
Grow Old and Wise.
Leave Your Money to Someone
You Love Who Loves You Back.

DIE IN YOUR SLEEP.

Sharon Esther Lampert
Poet, Philosopher, Prophet, Peacemaker, Pin-Up, Prodigy
www.WorldFamousPoems.com
FANS@SharonEstherLampert.com

CPSIA information can be obtained
at www.ICGtesting.com
Printed in the USA
LVHW060829010522
717347LV00025B/328

9 781885 872821